THE NAIL IN
HEALTH AND DISEASE

THE NAIL IN HEALTH AND DISEASE

Nardo Zaias, M.D.
Miami Beach, Florida

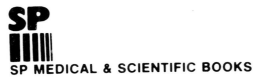

SP MEDICAL & SCIENTIFIC BOOKS

New York

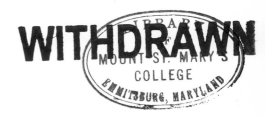

SPECTRUM PUBLICATIONS, INC.
175-20 Wexford Terrace, Jamaica, New York 11432

Library of Congress Cataloging in Publication Data

Zaias, Nardo.
  The nail.

  Includes index.
  1. Nails (Anatomy)—Diseases. 2. Nails
(Anatomy) I. Title.
RL165.Z34   616.5'47   78–18238
ISBN 0-89335-066-4

Acknowledgments

In his air-conditioned office, Dr. G. Matoltsy spoke softly to the two of us, third-year residents in Miami. Marvin Lutzner and I had to choose subjects that could be studied presently and could lay the foundation for our future dermatologic academic careers. The choices, after the twenty-minute chat, were narrowed to two:

1. A reevaluation of the developmental stages of the skin adnexa, including ultrastructure, with the use of the newly installed prize of Dr. Harvey Blank's department, an RCA EM-38 electron microscope; and

2. The other subject, simply referred to as "THE NAIL."

I am indebted to Marvin Lutzner's lightning reply, choosing the adnexa that day in 1960, for starting my interest in "THE NAIL."

Fidel Castro provided further impetus in keeping my interest on the nail by having Dr. Pardo-Castello reside permanently, until his death, in Miami and at the University of Miami Department of Dermatology. His encouragement culminated in my presentation in 1961 at the American Academy of Dermatology—the embryology of the human nail.

Albert Kligman's superb and stimulating teaching conferences solidly cemented my future interest in the nail.

I am also indebted to all the colleagues who began to refer patients with nail problems from which I amassed the material I studied under the auspices of my chairman, Harvey Blank, at the University of Miami Medical School.

In addition, I have had the cooperation of many dermatologists, in particular, Drs. F. Ronchese, Robert Baran and Orville Stone, who have allowed me to use their clinical photographs of nail disorders.

Finally, I am greatful to the National Institutes of Health for their support.

An apology is forthcoming to the original describers of interesting syndromes and nail abnormalities. In the majority of cases, the most recent, complete review reference, and not the original, is used on the subject matter.

N.Z.
Miami Beach, 1980

Preface

The primary intent of this book is to familiarize the medical practitioner with the "nail unit" in a way which will render, correctly and more easily, the diagnosis of nail diseases. At the same time, it serves to encourage the treatment and corrective measures of the abnormalities, if possible, based on anatomical and physiological knowledge.

The chapters on anatomy, regeneration, and nail formation are basic to the author's intent. The content of the references quoted represents information which is proven and *not* controversial material. In addition, my own material not previously published is included.

I would like to introduce the anatomical concept that the *nail unit* consists of four different epithelial structures, each with its own characteristics, yet all interrelated. These four constituents are the Proximal Nail Fold (PNF), the Matrix (M), the Nail Bed (NB) and the Hyponychium (HYP). A disease may occur in any number of or all nail unit structures. A clear understanding of the anatomy, histology, and tissue kinetics of each constituent will be necessary and is the key factor in interpreting the abnormal findings of each of these constituents as disease occurs. It follows, therefore, that treatment and corrective measures should include the knowledge of not only the nail but also of its relationship to the bony phalanx and the digit.

Thus, on seeing the clinical nail signs, focus at the site of origin, and do not be confused by the signs of the end result of the disease. Also, the reader can then have a chronological appreciation as to when and for how long the disease has occurred and is continuing.

It is also the intent of the author to compile as many facts about human as well as animal nails and claws so that this may be used as a reference text.

Contents

CHAPTER 1

Anatomy and Physiology

The "nail plate" on the dorsum of all fingers and toes shapes and greatly enhances the coordinated fine digital movements. Four differently keratinizing epithelial structures make up the nail unit. What is commonly termed the nail (nail plate) is the horny end product of the most important epithelial component, the matrix.

The nail plate is a roughly rectangular, transparent/translucent, flat, horny structure which moves with the horny layer of the nail bed to extend unattached as a "free edge" growing past the distal tip of the finger. The normally pink nail bed (its color is due to an enriched vascular network) is seen through the transparent nail plate (Fig. 1). Usually in the thumbs and commonly in other fingers and large toenails, a whitish, crescent-shaped "lunula" is seen extending from under the proximal nail fold (Figs. 1, 2, 3, 4). Thus there are two lateral and one proximal nail folds.

Looking at the thumb's profile, the reader will notice that the nail plate emerges from under the proximal nail fold at an angle to the surface of the dorsum of digit skin (Fig. 5). This angle, commonly referred to as Lovibond's angle,[1] should always be less than 180°. Only in abnormal states, e.g., clubbing, is this emergence angle greater than 180° (see Chapter 23).

Each nail component (Fig. 1)—the proximal nail fold (PNF), the matrix (M), the nail bed (NB) and the hyponychium (HYP)—is an epithelial structure, like skin and hair, having an epidermis with a "live" germinative cell layer that differentiates and becomes the horny layer, or end product, which is considered "dead." These four components can easily be differentiated histologically from each other and can be traced as the nail unit develops embryologically (see Chapter 4).

COMPONENTS OF THE NAIL

The Proximal Nail Fold (PNF)

This is an extension of the skin of surface fingers and toes which becomes a fold and lies superficial to the matrix, which is deeper in the finger and toe substance (Figs. 3, 6;

chapter 4. It has two epithelial borders, a superficial and a deep layer. Only the superficial layer can be seen from the exterior. The cuticle, the horny layer of the PNF, "rides" adherent on the surface of the nail plate for a short distance before being shed normally or cut away by a manicurist (Fig. 13). The superficial PNF layer is like the epidermis elsewhere but has its own characteristics; i.e., the skin distally from the distal interphalangeal joint to the nail plate is devoid of hair follicles and finger print pattern, and is thinner than the dorsum of digit skin (Fig. 2). An occasional sweat gland may be seen proximally rather than distally. Often visible (at the tip of the PNF) are capillary loops described as hallmarks of certain disease states, e.g., lupus erythematosus, dermatomyositis and phototoxic conditions; however, these capillary loops may be seen normally.

Histology

The ventral PNF skin is thinner than its superficial counterpart and appears not to have marked epidermal ridges. In this respect, it shows similarities with the eyelids and scrotal skin. It may be the portal of entry of irritating as well as allergic chemicals which may be causative in a complex environment-influenced set of circumstances in the disease known as chronic paronychia. The ventral PNF layer is continuous with the matrix epithelium. These can be differentiated by observing that the PNF has a granular layer while the matrix does not. The arrows in Figs. 7 and 8 are positioned at the junction of these structures (Figs. 3, 6, 7 and 8).

The Matrix (M)

Deeper in the substance of the digits is the most important of the nail unit constitutents, located millimeters from the dorsal mid-portion of the distal bony phalanx (Fig 6). The matrix epithelium is bordered proximally by the ventral PNF and distally by the nail bed (Figs. 13, 15). The pattern of its epithelial rete is rootlike and seems to have a firm attachment to its dermal papillary counterpart (Figs. 7, 8, 9). The histologic observations of the firm attachment of the matrix epithelium to the dermis are excellently described by Hashimoto.[2] The matrix basal cells have small villous structures which project into the dermis (Fig. 10, arrows down). From these basal cell projections, anchoring filaments are seen to form bundles which extend (arrow) from the basement membrane (BM) to collagen fibers in the dermis (arrow sets, Fig. 11). By light microscopy, the epithelial differentiation process is similar to that seen in the hair matrix. The end product, or horny layer, the nail plate is considered a "hard keratinous" structure.

Histology—The Differentiation Process

The matrix epithelium consists of basal cells which seem to have their vertical axis directed diagonally/distally, resulting in the nail's growing out rather than up from under the PNF (Figs. 9, 12; see Chapter 4). As they differentiate, matrix basaloid cells (Figs. 8, 9, 12) flatten their nuclei, which begin to fragment and take on a more eosinophilic cytoplasm; thus the keratogenous zone is formed (Figs. 9, 12). The cells lose most of the nuclear materials and nail plate cells, or onychocytes are formed. Nuclear fragments (Fig. 12) may be detected by DNA stains in the well-formed nail plate a considerable distance from the matrix, but these disappear completely nearing the distal free edge. This implies that DNA-ases, as well as RNA-ases, are still operational in the "dead, horny end product." This is unique to the nail plate. It also explains the earlier observation by Mitchell[3] of why leukonychial spots, parakeratonic foli, which usually follow matrix trauma such as manicuring, are reduced in the surface area and may totally disappear by the time they reach the free edge of the nail plate. The matrix does not exhibit a keratonyaline granular layer. The nail plate is transparent, does not take eosin, but is strongly basic Fuchsin–positive (acid-fast positive).

The Lunula

Returning to the thumb, we observe the lunula (half-moon) to be whitish and opaque (Fig. 1, 3). As stated previously, the lunula is the most distal area of the matrix. Since it is the only visible area of the matrix, we must assume that the whole matrix is opaque white (Fig. 13). Not all fingers exhibit a lunula; most consistently, it is seen in the thumb and index finger (Figs. 2, 3). Cerebral hemispheric dominançe (handedness) can be ascertained by a greater surface area of the lunula and nail plate of dominant thumb.[4,5]

Color. Many investigators have written about the whitish color of the lunula, but none has presented convincing data. Various facts are noted and may play a role in the explanation of the whitish appearance (Fig. 13):

(1) The nail plate is very transluscent and almost transparent. This results in a "pink" appearance to the nail bed as light going through the nail plate reflects off the vasculature of the nail bed (Fig. 13).

(2) The nail plate over the lunula (distal matrix) is thinner than over the nail bed.

(3) The whitish color of the lunula coincides with the presence and shape of the keratogenous zone (KZ) of the matrix. In this zone there is nuclear retention

(4) Accounts of a reduced vasculature supplying the matrix have been disproven by this author.

At a glance, it would seem that the whitish color of the lunula is produced by the same phenomenon of light diffraction that occurs in the distal free edge of the nail, onycholytic nails, leukonychial spots secondary to manipulation of the matrix, and proximal nail fold. In the lunula, the KZ cells (in themselves a denser object) appear whitish, exactly like leukonychial spots (white spots) a parakeratolic focus of onychocytes.

The lunula plays an important role in shaping the nail plate. This was demonstrated by Clark LeGros[6] (Fig. 14).

In addition, the lunula is the portion of the matrix to first differentiate during developmental times (see Chapter 2) (Fig. 17).

Thus it makes sense that the configuration of the genetically predetermined nail area (lunula) shapes the free edge of the nail plate. Failure to reconstruct the lunula's shape during trauma or during surgical intervention may result in nail plate dystrophy.

Melanocytes

In the Negro race, melanocytes normally are abundant in the matrix epithelium. The color of the nail plate varies from very light to very dark gray. Generally, the nail plate may pigment diffusely, but longitudinal bands of pigment are often seen. These represent foci of melanocytic hyperplasia and are not nevi (see Chapter 2).

The Nail Bed (NB)

The nail bed is defined as that area of the nail unit beginning at the lunula (Figs. 1, 2, 3, 6, 13, 15) and extending to the hyponychium (Figs. 3, 6, 18, 21). Most of the surface of the dorsum of the fingertip is covered by the nail bed. It has two characteristic features: (1) its epidermis and (2) the spatial arrangement of its epidermal and dermal ridges. The nail bed consists of epidermal ridges, not rete, aligned longitudinally and almost parallel to each other. These ridges extend from the lunula distally (Fig. 21) to the hyponychium and fit tongue-and-groove fashion between similarly arranged dermal ridges (Fig. 16, arrows up and down). The appearance of the nail bed after the removal of the nail plate (Fig. 19) suggests the effect of the fingerprint pattern (Fig. 20). It can easily be seen that small blood vessels along these dermal ridges (Figs. 16, 17, 19) affected by either disease processes or trauma are responsible for the so-called splinter hemorrhages known only to occur in the nail bed. The architecture of the dermal/epidermal relationship in the lateral margins of the nail bed shows more complex primary epidermal ridges with secondary smaller ridges (Fig. 17).

The epidermis of the nail bed is unique in that by light microscopy examination there is an obvious lack of mitosis in the basal cells and also in that the horny cell layer is scanty. The differentiation of the epidermis is similar to that of the inner root sheath of hair. As basal cells differentiate to the surface of the epidermis (Figs. 16, 17), they lose their nuclei and become nail bed horn cells. There is no granular layer visible by light microscopy; however, Hashimoto[2] has described a keratohyline granular zone in the normal nail bed of embryonic fingers 17 weeks in development (through electron microscopy). In disease states, a rich granular layer involving the nail bed is not infrequent. The horny layer of the nail bed is scant. Few horn cells are added to the underside of the nail plate. The nail horn cells stain eosinophilic in contrast to the unstained nail plate cells (Figs. 16, 17). The cells of the basal layer of the nail bed epidermis "move" from an area near the lunula to the hyponychium. On the way, some of these cells differentiate distally and result in horn cells all along the nail bed epidermis. This "movement" takes place at the same rate as nail plate growth (see Chapter 4).

Not uncommonly, fairly large epithelial buds have been seen in the nail bed and matrix and recently have been reported by Lewin.[7] These consist of solid outpocketing of basal cells which show no abnormalities. Melanocytes normally are not found in the nail bed epithelium but may occur in the Negro race and, rarely, in Orientals.

The Hyponychium (HYP)

The hyponychium is the most distal nail unit component, extending from the nail bed and terminating at the distal groove (Figs. 3, 6, 18, 21). The epidermis making up the hyponychium is similar to plantar and volar epidermis. Its epidermal rete pattern is similar to that of palmar and plantar epidermis, as is its dermis papillary pattern. The gross hyponychium normally is not seen but can be observed in fingers of nail biters. Rarely, a congenital "extended hyponychium" is seen[8] (Fig. 22); this has also been reported and termed pterygium inversum unguis.[9,10] The stratum corneum of the hyponychium normally is seen accumulating under the distal free edge of the nail plate. The distal groove seems more prominent in fingers. A wide groove separates the hyponychium from the volar skin (Figs. 3, 6). In primates and lower animals, the distal groove may be very prominent. In the microbiologic disease states, the hyponychial horny layer is the portal of entry to the nail unit (see Chapters 8, 15).

THE DERMIS

The dermal component of the nail unit is unique in that it is limited by the underlying phalanx and there is no subcutaneous tissue. In the matrix area, the dermal architecture is classical with papillae accommodating the arbor-like ridges of the matrix (Figs. 7, 21). In the nail bed epidermal ridges (described previously and seen in Figs. 16, 17, 21) harbor the fine capillaries which, when disrupted, result in splinter hemorrhages commonly seen in normal and disease states. Specialized vascular tissues are also present in the digits. The glomus is one of these structures, particularly in the nail bed[11] (Fig. 15). In clubbed fingers, dense fibrovascular hyperplasis of the nail bed and particularly under the matrix is responsible for the characteristic exaggerated angle of the nail plate (Figs. 2, 6). The capillaries of the proximal fold have been studied extensively by capillary microscopy and attempts to diagnose various disease states by the pattern of these capillaries have been generally unsuccessful. Some capillary loops normally are seen at the proximal nail fold, but in general these are observed in disease states such as lupus erythematosus, scleroderma and dermatomyositis.[12] The connective tissue of the nail unit consists mostly of reticular dermis as well as ligaments and bone-associated connective tissue. There is no subcutaneous fat of deep dermis between the phalanx and the nail unit. Nerve endings and nerve trunks are also numerous, with specialized nerve structures such as Vater-Pacini corpuscles and Meissner corpuscles; however, these are noted to be more at the fingertip of the phalanx. There are no adnexal structures arising from the nail bed or hyponychium.

ULTRASTRUCTURE

The ultrastructure of the nail is known from relatively few studies. Hashimoto and associates[13,14] have described various embryo nail unit constituents (matrix, nail bed, etc.). Yet I cannot agree with the concepts formulated from these studies, e.g., the use of terms such as the dorsal nail matrix when reference is being made to the ventral component of the proximal nail fold and other new unwarranted terminology.

According to Hashimoto, the keratinization process of the human toenail plate cells from nail matrix was found to be identical with that of epidermal stratum corneum cells, particularly in the formation of the marginal band, or broad zone, and in the discharge of the membrane-coating granules (MCG's) that form the intercellular cement. However, MCG's were not responsible for additions to the broad zone. The most striking difference between the keratinization of the nail plate cells and epidermal stratum corneum cells is that in the nail the keratin fibrils (or keratin pattern) form by accretions of cytoplasmic filaments without the formation of keratohyaline granules. In this respect, the nail is identical with hair cortex.

Structures similar to MCG's were described by Matoltsky[15] from abnormal nail plate. The adult matrix of toenails has also been studied by Hashimoto.[16] Caputo and Dadati[17] studied the nail plate after treatment with thioglycolic acid. The authors concluded:)1) "The cell's cytoplasm consists of keratin fibrils combining in bundles and immersed in a nonstructural amorphous mass. These bundles lay in no precise direction but are arranged haphazardly within the cell," and (2) "The intercellular links, which are quantitatively numerous may present three aspects: (a) the tight junction, that is, complete contact between two opposite membranes, (b) intermediate junction type, that is, the space between the two membranes is unconstant (200–300A) and a dense nonhemogenous substance can be observed within it, separated from the cell membranes by two thin light bands, and (c) desmosone-like type with fibrillar bundles which converge toward the cell membrane. However, the typical stratification after cementing substance is missing from these bonds."

These studies have not been able to confirm that there are three distinct layers on the nail plate. Scanning electron microscopy of the nail plate by Forslind and Thyrasson[18] differentiated a hard dorsal nail plate and a more plastic intermediate nail plate. The authors, however, did not realize that a section taken vertically through the nail plate is made up of cells of different ages: a much older superficial nail plate layer and a more recent lower layer of the nail plate. The nail plate is formed as a sheet from the apex of the matrix to the lunula, and the superficial layers are therefore produced by the apex cells while the lowermost layers of the nail plate are produced by the lunula. Thus, at a vertical cut, an older (earlier-produced nail plate) is present with a younger (later-produced) nail plate.

GROWTH

The nail plate consists of dead, cornified cells produced by the matrix. The basal-like cells of the matrix lose their nuclei, flatten and cornify, and are added to the already formed solid nail plate. The rate of growth of the nail plate is determined by the turnover rate of the matrix cells. Shortly after death, matrix cells do not incorporate tritiated thymidine in their nuclei and appear to be incapable of DNA synthesis and cell division; therefore, the nail does not grow. Previous observations relating nail growth after death were, in fact, erroneously reporting apparent growth caused by the severe post-mortem drying and shrinking of the soft tissues around the nail plate.

Fingernails grow faster than toenails. Nails of individual fingers of the same hand grow at different rates.[19] The average growth of the thumbnail is 0.10–0.12 mm daily. The rate growth is thought to be greater in the second to third decades with a slight decline thereafter.[20] Family tendencies favoring similar growth rates among individuals have been noted,[21] as well as increased growth during the summer and diminished growth in cold climates[22] (Fig. 23). Many systemic disorders affect nail growth by deceleration, and many manifest by thinning and grooving of the nail plate. This phenomenon is best appreciated weeks after the event has occurred. Acute viral infection states, such as mumps and measles, are most often reported to affect nails. Starvation has also been associated with reduction of nail growth. Increase in growth rate can be seen during pregnancy,[23] nail biting trauma[24] and regrowth after avulsion (Fig. 24).

The ingestion of gelatin has not been conclusively shown to specifically encourage nail growth or nail strength.

CHEMICAL COMPOSITION AND BIOCHEMISTRY

Little is known about the chemistry and biochemistry of nails. Earlier investigators studied mainly total contents of various organic and mineral components of normal as well as specific diseased nails. A brief listing is presented for reference (see Table I): sulfur;[25] total nonprotein nitrogen; urea nitrogen; ammonia nitrogen; uric acid[26] in gout; creatinine[26,27] in chronic renal failure; sodium[28] elevated in cystic fibrosis despite normal values in sweat; calcium elevated in older normals[29] and in traumatic states,[30] not abnormal in brittle nails;[31] phosphorus; zinc; magnesium; manganese; silicon; lead; boron; titanium; strontium; silver; aluminum;[29] copper,[29] elevated in Wilson's disease;[31-33] iron,[34] cholesterol,[35] and sulfhydryl-disulfide groups have demonstrated in the nail. In early embryonic life, there is a very high concentration of sulfhydryl groups;[36] this concentration decreases as the fetus reaches the newborn age and stabilizes at about age three.[37] Disulfide groups are present in small amounts in embryonic nails and rapidly increase as term and infancy approach.[36,37]

Iron is also found in higher amounts in infants' nails as compared to those of 40- to 70-year-olds. During the 20th to 40th years, the amount of iron is less than during the 40th to 70th years. (These levels were determined colorimetrically.) In cystic fibrosis of the pancreas, abnormally higher levels of calcium, magnesium and sodium have been reported to reflect more accurately a homozygous patient than the sodium level alone.[38] Ungulic acid, a new ganglioside sulfate, has been isolated from the horse hoof.[39]

Recently, Baden[40] and colleagues have presented data concerning certain biochemical events related to nails and compared them to hair and stratum corneum.

From x-ray diffraction and electron microscopy studies, Forslind[18] relates the hardness of nails to cell arrangement, cell adhesion, and ultrastructure arrangement of the keratin fibrils.

Table I
Mineral Elements in Normal and Diseased Nail

	Neutron dosimetry (mg/gm NAIL)	
Aluminum	0.00000000045[29]	
Antimony		
Arsenic	[41]	Poisoning[47]
Boron	0.007–0.006[29]	
Bromine	[41]	
Calcium	0.671–0.806[29,44]	
	3.64 ± 1.77[28a]	9.96 ± 3.70 Cystic fibrosis[38a]
		Kwashiakor[48a]
Copper	0.029–0.089[29,44,45]	
Gold	0.00044 ± 0.0006[41,44]	
Iron	0.029–0.064[29,34]	**30b**
Lead	0.0097–0.024[29]	
Magnesium	0.1–0.121[29,44]	
	3.45 ± 1.5[38a]	4.72 ± 1.45 Cystic fibrosis[38a]
		Kwashiakor[48a]
Manganese	0.002 ± 0.001[29,45,46]	
Phosphorus	0.00008–0.00027[29]	
Potassium		Kwashihkor[48c]
Silicon	0.17–0.54[29]	
Silver	0.0000000048[29]	
Sodium	2.4 ± 1.8[41,45]	
	3.34 ± 1.4[38]	9.12–3.20 Cystic fibrosis[38c]
		Kwashiakor[48c]
Strontium	0.00000016[29]	
Sulfur	36.6 ± 2.1[42,43]	
Titanium	0.0000016[29]	
Zinc	0.106–0.154[29,41,44,49]	

[a]Fluorometrically
[b]Colormetrically
[c]Flame photometry

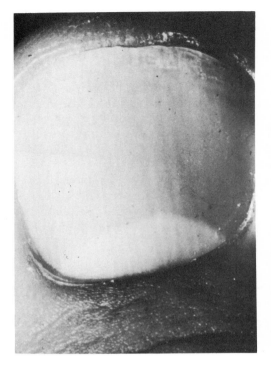

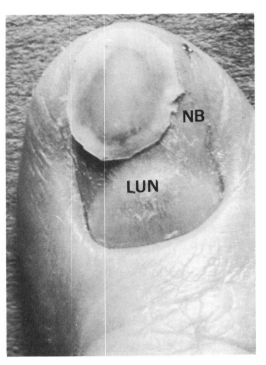

Fig. 1. Normal fingernail showing whitish lunula, pink nail bed.

Fig. 2. Thumbnail. Nail plate remains as island attached to underlying nail bed. Lunula (LUN) can be seen as whitish, opaque structure. Nail bed (NB). Note lateral and proximal nail fold.

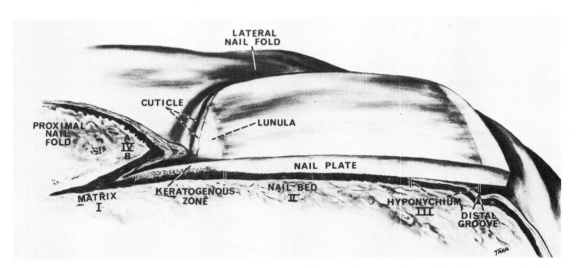

Fig. 3. Diagrammatic drawing of longitudinal section of fingernail showing four epithelial components: (1) matrix, (2) nail bed, (3) hyponychium, (4) proximal nail fold. (N. Zaias, *Arch. Derm.* 87: 37-53, 1963)

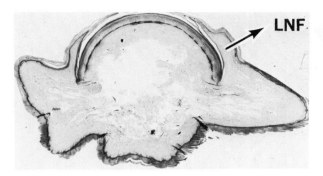

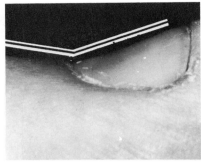

Fig. 4. Cross-section of finger at level of nail bed. Note lateral nail folds (LNF). H&E X12.

Fig. 5. Skin of proximal nail fold (PNF) should be on angle less than 180° with the emerging nail plate.

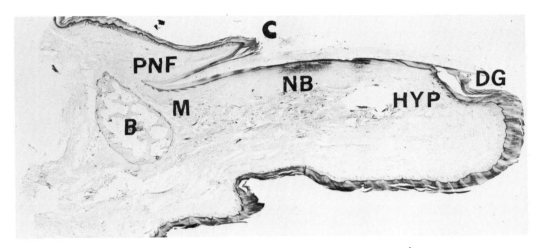

Fig. 6. Longitudinal section of fingernail. Note proximity of bone (B) to matrix (M) and that the cuticle (C), is the stratum corneum of the proximal nail fold (PNF). Note also that the distal groove (DG) exists in humans. H&E X12.

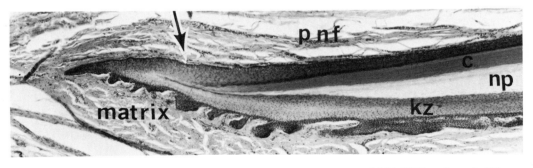

Fig. 7. Close-up from Fig. 6 of matrix area in which junction of proximal nail fold (PNF) and matrix (M) can be seen (arrow). Note rootlike epidermal rete of matrix. Keratogenous zone is seen. Nail plate (NP), cuticle (C). H&E X40. (N. Zaias, *Arch. Derm. 99:* 569, 1969)

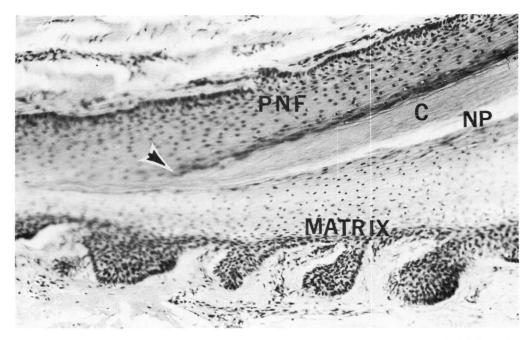

Fig. 8. Close-up of Fig. 7, (arrow) showing border of proximal nail fold (PNF) with matrix (M) (arrow). Granular layer of proximal nail fold epithelium disappears as matrix begins. Cuticle (C), nail plate (NP). H&E X150.

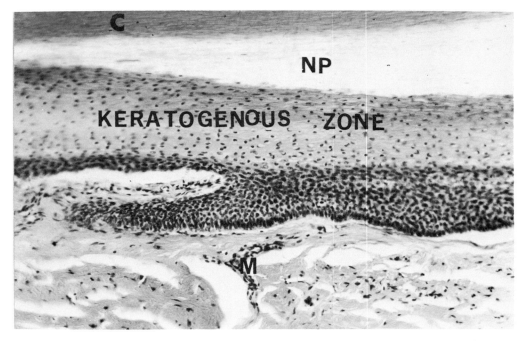

Fig. 9. Close-up of matrix in Fig. 7, near keratogenous zone (KZ), showing basal cells of matrix flattening or to becoming transparent nail plate (NP) cells, which do not take hematoxylin stain. H&E X140.

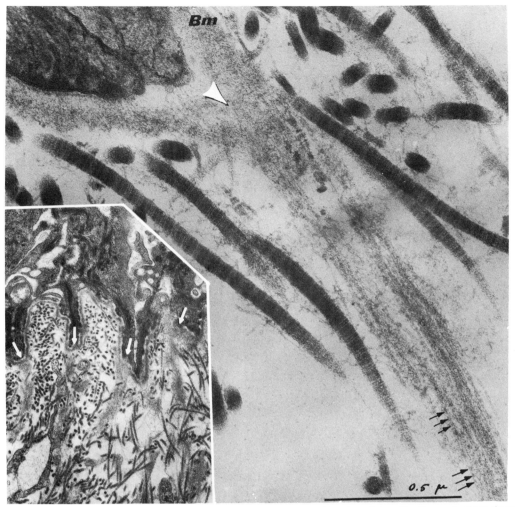

Fig. 10. Low-power electromicrograph of matrix showing basilar projections (arrows down) into dermis. X13,250.

Fig. 11. Higher magnification of tip of basilar projections showing attachment of fibrillar bundles from basement membrane (BM) (arrows) to collagen fibers. X109,500. (Courtesy K. Hashimoto, *J. Inv. Derm. 56:* 237, 1971)

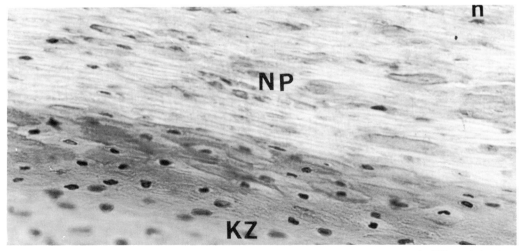

Fig. 12. Close-up of keratogenous zone (KZ) in Fig. 9, showing nucleated cells of matrix differentiating into nail plate cells (NP), which are devoid of nuclei. Some nuclei (N) remain for short distance in nail plate. H&E X400.

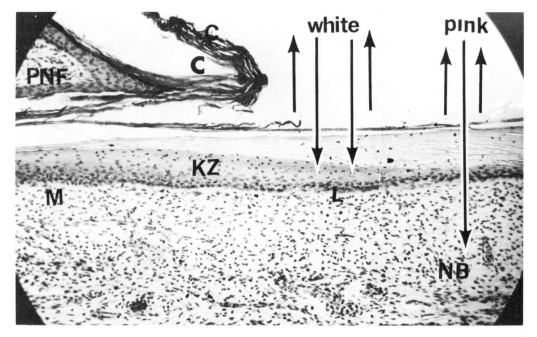

Fig. 13. Longitudinal section of human finger in which lunula (L) is demonstrated as distal portion of matrix (M), extending from under proximal nail fold (PNF), and is seen grossly as whitish area. Keratogenous zone (KZ). Nail bed (NB) grossly is pink. H&E X120.

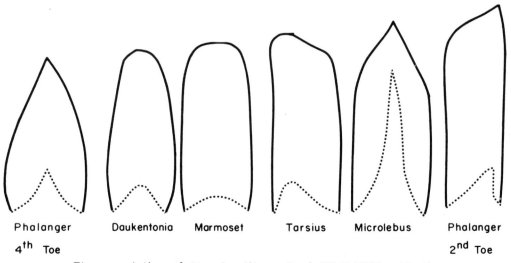

Phalanger   Daukentonia   Marmoset   Tarsius   Microlebus   Phalanger
4th Toe   2nd Toe

The correlation of the claw like nail of PRIMATES with the shape of the lunula.

Fig. 14. Shape of lunula correlates with shape of nail plate.

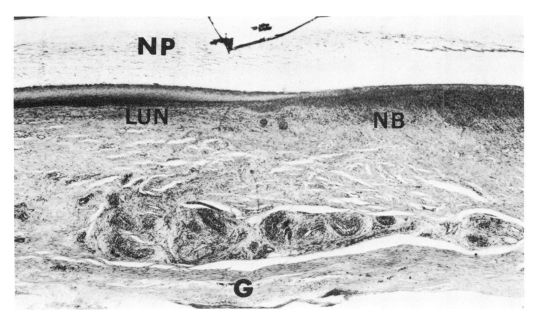

Fig. 15. Longitudinal section at lunula (LUN)/nail bed (NB) junction. Grossly, nail plate (NP) has been incized at end of lunula. Note presence of glomus (G) and vascular bodies in dermis. H&E X120. (N. Zaias, *Arch. Derm. 99*: 169, 1969)

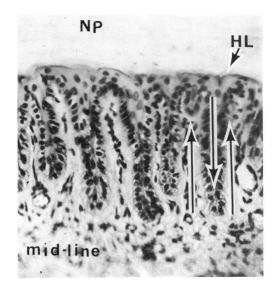

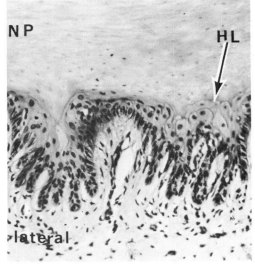

Fig. 16. Cross-section of nail bed, showing nail bed epidermal rete as long ridges interlacing with similar dermal ridges. Horny later (HL) of nail stains lightly eosinophilic. Nail plate (NP). H&E X450. (N. Zaias, *Arch. Derm. 99*: 369, 1969)

Fig. 17. Cross-section of lateral aspects of nail bed showing rootlike epithelial rete resulting in strong attachment of nail bed to underlying dermis. Nail plate (NP), horny layer (HL).

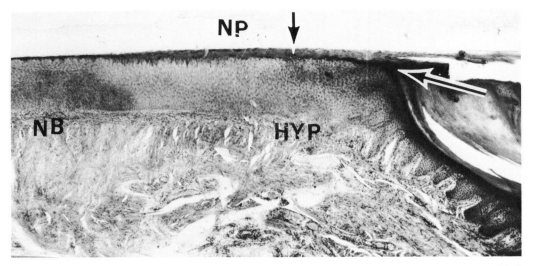

Fig. 18. Longitudinal section of nail bed (NB) hyponychium relationship showing hyponychium as a modified extension of volar epidermis and distinguishable from nail bed by lack of granular layer in its epidermal structure (arrow down). Horizontal arrow demarcates stratum corneum of HYP and distal groove. Portal of entry of microbiologic agents in onychomycosis and onycholysis. (N. Zaias, *Arch. Derm. 99*: 370, 1969)

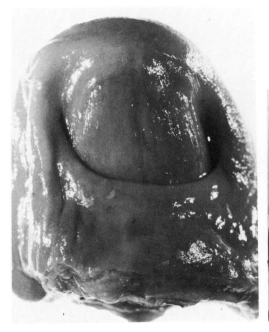

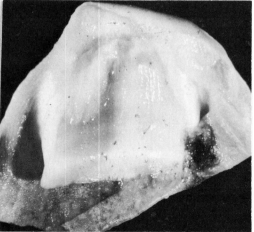

Fig. 19. Special preparation of toenail unit in which epithelial structures have been separated from underlying dermis by heat. Note lateral and proximal nail folds, as well as dermal pattern.

Fig. 20. Underside of epithelial structures of toenail unit removed from Fig. 16, showing nail bed longitudinal epidermal "rete."

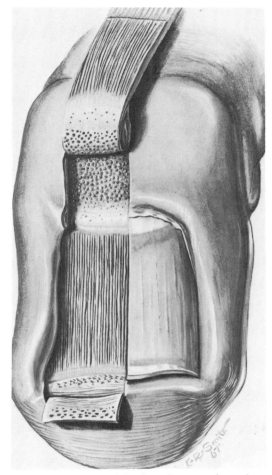

Fig. 21. Drawing of the dermal topography underlying nail unit. Note dermal papillae of matrix, the
dermal ridges of nail bed and dermal papillae of hyponychium. Anatomic pathology of splinter hemorrhages is obvious. (N. Zaias, *Arch. Derm. 107*: 193,
1973)

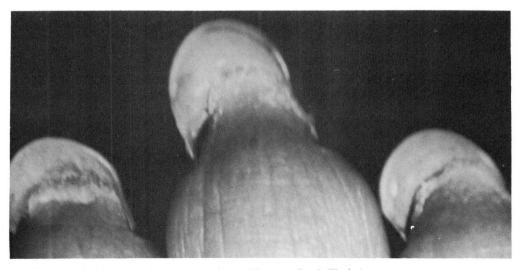

Fig. 22. Normal variant. Prominent hyponychium. (Courtesy Dr. J. Ziegler)

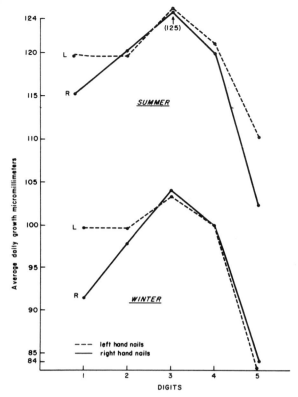

Fig. 23. Nail growth in summer appears to be increased as compared to that in winter; middle finger nail growth appears to be increased over other nails of same hand. (LeGros & Buxton, *Brit. J. Derm. 50*: 121, 1938)

Fig. 24. During pregnancy, greatest nail growth rate appears to be just prior to delivery, with rapid decrease of growth post-partum. (Hewitt & Hillman, *Am. J. Clin. Nutr.* 436, 1966)

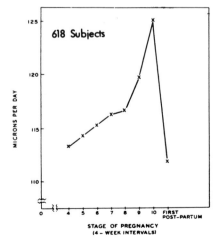

NOTES

1. Lovibond, J.L.: Diagnosis of clubbed fingers. *Lancet 1*: 363-364, 1938.
2. Hashimoto, K., Gross, B.G., Nelson, R., and Lever, W.F.: Ultrastructure of the skin of human embryos. III. The formation of the nail on 16–18 week old embryos. *J. Inv. Derm. 47*: 205-217, 1966.
3. Mitchell, J.C.: A clinical study of leuconychia. *Brit. J. Derm. 65*: 125-130, 1953.
4. Block, J.E.: Thumbs down on left handedness. *N. Eng. J. Med. 29*: 307, 1975.
5. Pittsley, R.A., and Shearn, M.A.: Nail down handedness. *JAMA 236*: 819, 1976.
6. LeGros Clark, W.B.: The problems of the claw in primates. *Proc. Zool. Soc. 1*: 1-24, 1936.
7. Lewin, K: The normal fingernail. *Brit. J. Derm. 77*: 421-430, 1965.
8. Odom, R.B., Stein, K.M., and Maibach, H.I.: Congenital painful aberrant hyponychium. *Arch. Derm. 110*: 89-90, 1974.
9. Caputo, R., and Prandi, G.: Pterygium inversum unguis. *Arch. Derm. 108*: 817-818, 1973.
10. Patterson, J.W. Pterygium inversum unguis-like changes in scleroderma. *Arch. Derm. 113:* 1429–1430, 1977.
11. Hale, A.R., and Brucn, G.E.: The arteriovenous anastomoses and blood vessels of the human finger. *Med. 39*: 191-240, 1960.
12. Ross, J.B.: Nail fold capillaroscopy, a useful aid in the diagnosis of collagen vascular disease. *J. Inv. Derm. 47*: 282-285, 1966.
13. Hashimoto, K.: Ultrastructure of the human toenail. II. *J. Ultrastructure Res. 36*: 391-410, 1971.
14. Hashimoto, K.: Ultrastructure of the human toenail cell migration, keratinization and formation of the intercellular cement. *Arch. Derm. Forsch 240*: 1-22, 1971.
15. Matoltsy, A.G., and Matoltsy, M.N.: Cytoplasmic droplets of pathologic horny cells. *J. Invest. Derm. 38*: 323-325, 1962.
16. Hashimoto, K.: Ultrastructure of the human toenail. I. Proximal nail matrix. *J. Inv. Derm. 56:* 235-246, 1971.
17. Caputo, R., and Dadati, E.: Preliminary observations about the ultrastructure of the human nail plate treated with thioglycolic acid. *Arch. Clin. Exp. Derm. 231*: 344-354, 1968.
18. Forslind, B., and Thyrasson, N.: On the structure of the normal nail: a scanning electromicroscopy study. *Arch. Derm. Forsch 251*: 199-204, 1975.
19. LeGros Clark, W.B., Buxton, L.H., and Dudley, P.: Studies in nail growth. *Brit. J. Derm. & Syph. 50*: 221-235, 1938.
20. Bean, W.B.: Nail growth: a twenty year study. *Arch. Int. Med. 111*: 476-482, 1963.
21. Hamilton, J.B., Terada, H., and Mestler, G.E.: Studies of growth throughout the life span in Japanese; growth and size of nails and their relationship to age, sex, hereditary and other factors. *J. Gerontology 10*: 401-415, 1955.
22. Goeghegan, B., Robert, D.F., and Sampford, M.R.: A possible climatic effect on nail growth. *J. Appl. Physiol. 13*: 135-138, 1958.
23. Hewitt, D., add Hillman, R.: Relation between rate of nail growth in pregnant women and estimated previous general growth rate. *Am. J. Clin. Nutrition 19*: 436, 1966.
24. LeGros Clark, W.B., and Buxton, L.H.: Studies in nail growth. *Brit. J. Derm. 50*: 221-235, 1938.
25. Klauder, J.V. and Brown, H.: Sulphur content of hair and nails in abnormal states. *Arch Derm. & Syph. 31*: 26-34, 1935.
26. Bolliger, A., and Gross, R.: Non-keratin of human toenails. *Austral. J. Exp. Biol. 31*: 127-130, 1953.
27. Levitt, J.I.: Creatinine concentration of human fingernail and toenail clippings; application in determining the duration of renal failure. *Ann. Int. Med. 64*: 312-327, 1953.
28. Kopito, L., Mahmoodian, A., Townley, R.R.W., Knaw, K.T., and Schwachman, M.: Studies in cystic fibrosis. *New Eng. J. Med. 272*: 504-509, 1965.
29. Goldblum, R.W., Derby, S.E., and Lerner, A.B.: The metal content of skin, nails and hair. *J. Invest. Derm. 20*: 13-18, 1953.
30. Blakey, P.R., Earland, C., Stell, J.G.P., and Swift. D.: Heterotopic calcification of human nail and hair. *Nature 207*: 190-191, 1965.
31. Kile, R.L.: Some mineral constituents of fingernails. *Arch. Derm. 70*: 75-83, 1954.
32. Rice, E.W., and Goldstein, N.P.: Copper content of hair and nails in Wilson's disease (hepatolenticular degeneration). *Metabolism 10*: 1085-1087, 1961.
33. Martin, S.M.: Copper content of hair and nails of normal individuals and of patients with hepatolenticular degeneration. *Nature 202*: 903-904, 1964.
34. Jacobs, A., and Jenkins, D.J.: The iron content of fingernails. *Brit. J. Derm. 72:* 145-148, 1960.
35. Hotta, K., and Takazi, K.: The cholesterol content of nails and hoofs of different animals. *J. Biochem. (Japan) 25*: 109, 1937.

36. Zaias, N.: Embryology of the human nail. *Arch. Derm. 87*: 37-53, 1963.

37. Knox et al.: The construction of sulphydryl and disulfide in human epidermis, hair and nails. *J. Invest. Derm. 38*: 69-75, 1962.

38. Leonard, P.J., and Morris, W.P.: Sodium, calcium, magnesium levels in nails of children with cystic fibrosis of the pancreas. *Arch. Dis. Child. 47*: 495-498, 1972.

39. Leikola, E., Nieminen, E., and Teppo, A.: New sialic acid containing sulfolipid-ungulic acid. *J. Lipid Res. 10*: 440-444, 1969.

40. Baden, H.P., Goldsmith, L.A., and Flemming, B.C.; A comparative study of the physiochemical properties of human keratinized tissue. *Biochem. Biophys. Acta 322:* 269-278, 1973.

41. Petuskov, A.A., Linckin, D.M., Ballius, J.F., and Brownell, G.L.: Determination of minerals. *J. Nuc. Med. 10*: 730, 1969.

42. Peterson, D.F., Michell, V.E., and Langham, W.H.: Determination of minerals. *Health Physics 6*: 1, 1961.

43. Amin, S.R., and Gupta, B.L.: Estimation of sulphur contact on human hair and nails for use in fast neutron dosimetry. *Health Physics 23*: 243-244, 1972.

CHAPTER 2

Embryology, Or Developmental Stages

A description and interpretation of the developmental stages of the human nail are presented in this chapter. Each nail unit component will be traced from its earliest developmental stages to its adult structure.

The earliest anatomical sign observed on the surface of the digit occurs at about 9 weeks in its development (Figs. 1, 2, 3). Grossly, a flattened rectangular area, known as the nail field, is outlined by grooves. These grooves are continuous and are the forerunners of the proximal, distal and lateral nail grooves. Later, as further development takes place, the nail field differentiates and forms all the nail unit structures which are barely recognizable in the gross specimen (Figs. 4–11). Changes occur in the entire finger and toe. As the digit elongates, its undifferentiated mesenchymal cells mature and differentiate into their respective adult structures (see figures of this chapter as summary). The epithelium covering the 9-week-old finger (Fig. 12) matures from a single layer or a few epithelial cells to a multilayer epithelium (Fig. 13). Activity is noted at the most proximal and distal areas of the nail field. There is also a distinct proliferative cell population, the basal cells, which begins to show a process of differentiation with the ultimate formation of "horn cells."

DISTAL NAIL FIELD—DEVELOPMENT OF THE NAIL BED AND HYPONYCHIUM

As can be seen, there are histological changes occurring in the most distal area of the nail field. This is first observed in the structure known as the distal ridge (DR) in fingers at about 11 weeks in development (Figs. 14, 15). More significantly, as the fetus grows older (Fig. 16), the epithelium of the nail field (future nail bed) begins to show both a granular and a horny layer starting distally and proceeding proximally (bent arrow down, Fig. 16; 20, 22). This event in itself is of interest since in the adult nail bed the epithelium does not exhibit a granular layer (light microscopically) unless it has been involved with trauma or disease.

At approximately 18 weeks of development (Figs. 23, 24, 26, 28), the embryonal nail bed epithelium begins to lose the granular zone which it previously exhibited. The granular zone seems to recede in a distal direction concomitantly with the movement distally of the formed nail plate (arrow down, Figs. 23, 26). This process can be followed in fingers of older fetuses (arrow down, Figs. 29, 32). The resulting nail bed, hyponychium and distal groove can be seen in the newborn (Figs. 36, 39).

PROXIMAL NAIL FIELD—THE MATRIX AND PROXIMAL NAIL FOLD

The earliest sign of the future nail unit is seen on the surface epithelium of the 9-week-old finger (Fig. 12). The arrow points to the border of histologically different epithelium. Distally from the arrow, the nail bed and hyponychium will develop. Proximally is the future proximal nail fold; at the arrow's point, the matrix will develop.

The 11-week-old nail field (Fig. 13) shows a wedge of cells arising from the proximal groove into the substance of the digit (arrow). This wedge of cells, termed the matrix primordium, will continue to grow diagonally/proximally until it reaches a distance of 1 millimeter from the bony phalanx in the full-term finger. The matrix primordium differentiates into two components as it matures. The superficial layer forms part of the future proximal nail fold epithelium (Figs. 14, 16, 17) and the deeper portions of the matrix primordium form the matrix epithelium. At 13 weeks in development, the nail matrix cells have differentiated from earlier matrix primordium cells and are producing the earliest nail plate seen in the most proximal nail field area (short single arrow, Fig. 16; arrow, Fig. 17; 18). The matrix primordium grows into the finger to produce a fully matured matrix cell population (Figs. 23, 24, 25, 29, 30, 32, 36). Thus the proximal nail fold is formed, lined with a dorsum of digit epithelium (Fig. 24).

That the first nail plate was formed in the lunula of the finger at age 12 to 13 weeks (Fig. 19) is demonstrated by the abundance of sulfhydryl radicals seen when these cells are stained (Figs. 19, 27). Subsequently, a more intense embryonal SH-positive nail plate (Figs. 31, 35) can be observed.

The matrix cells exhibit adult keratinization at age 20 weeks (Figs. 29, 38, 39). The earliest matrix cells, having now differentiated, form a nail plate which therefore moves distally (Figs. 29, 30, 32, 36). The nail plate eventually grows out over the nail bed and projects distally over the digit as a free edge, while its lateral borders are enveloped in the lateral nail fold (Figs. 33, 34, 37).

Table I
Approximate Age of Development at Which Various Structures Appear

Structure	Age
Nail field	9
Matrix primordium	11
Distal ridge (1st stratum corneum & granular layer)	11
Lunula (1st matrix & nail plate)	13
Cartilage	13
Bone	13
Epidermal rete	13
Sweat gland primordium	14
Sweat duct	15
Sweat gland	16

In the newborn, the nail plate is usually very long and bends volarly. This, however, represents the earliest attempt at nail plate formation and is very weak. With the nurse's cleaning of the newborn, the "early" plate immediately peels off.

Toes lag in formation by 4 weeks behind the corresponding fingers (Figs. 16, 21, 36, 40).

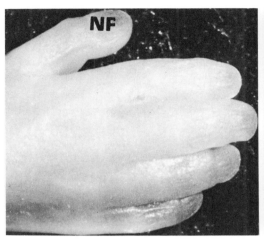

Fig. 1. Hand of 9-week-old human embryo showing flattened surfaces on dorsum of fingers, nail field (NF). X10.

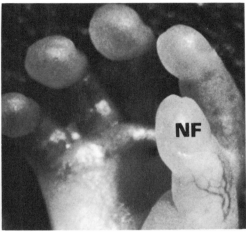

Fig. 2. Hand of 11-week-old embryo showing nail field (NF) clearly demarcated. X15.

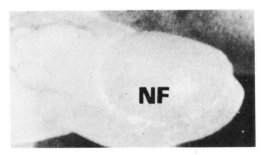

Fig. 3. Enlarged thumb of hand in Fig. 2 showing nail field (NF) clearly demarcated by proximal lateral and distal groves. X30.[1]

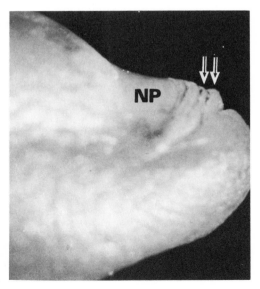

Fig. 4. Finger of 13-week-old embryo (lateral view) showing distal ridge (double arrow down), and proximal smooth surface of newly formed nail plate (NP). Distal groove can be seen distal to distal ridge. X20.

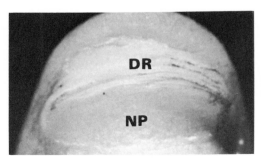

Fig. 5. Anterior/posterior view of finger in Fig. 4, showing same structures. X20.

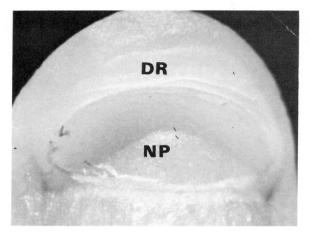

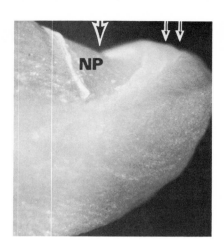

Fig. 6. Finger of 14-week-old embryo showing progression of newly formed nail plate (NP) and flattening of distal ridge. X20.

Fig. 7. Lateral view of finger in Fig. 6, showing flattening of distal ridge (double arrow) and developing nail plate (NP) (large arrow down). X20.[1]

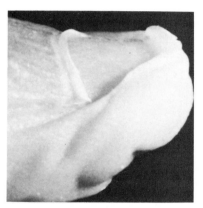

Fig. 8. Lateral view of 20-week-old embryo finger showing pronounced cuticle, nail plate and distal ridge in final stages. X10.

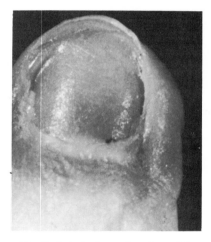

Fig. 9. Anterior/posterior view of finger in Fig. 8, X10.

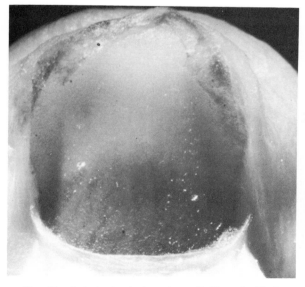

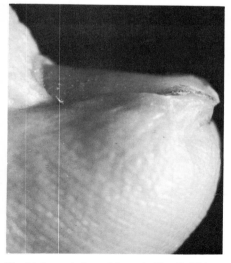

Fig. 10. Anterior/posterior view of 32-week-old finger showing nail plate (NP) barely extending past dorsum of fingertip as free edge. X20.

Fig. 11. Lateral view of finger in Fig. 10. X20.[1]

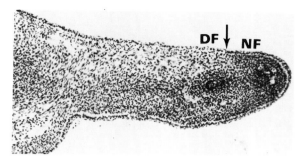

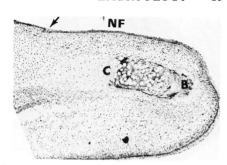

Fig. 12. Longitudinal section of thumb from 9-week-old finger showing undifferentiated mesenchymal cells with early differentiation of cartilage (C) in center finger. (Arrow down demarcates different types of embryonal epithelium. Nail field (NF) distal to arrow. Dorsum of finger epithelium (DF) proximal to arrow. H&E X120.

Fig. 13. Longitudinal section of thumb of 10-week-old finger showing more advanced differentiation of future phalanx, bone (B) and cartilage (C). Epithelium covering surface of finger is more developed and shows nail field (NF). H&E X120.[1]

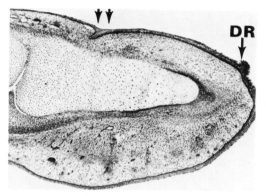

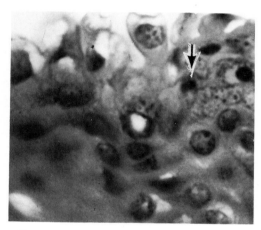

Fig. 14. Longitudinal section of 11-week-old finger showing nail field differentiating distally, with formation of distal ridge (DR) and proximally (double arrow) with formation of wedge of cells as precursor of matrix primordium. Epidermal rete and sweat gland anlage begin to form. H&E X120.[1]

Fig. 15. Higher magnification of distal ridge in Fig. 14, showing earliest keratohyaline granules. H&E X1600.

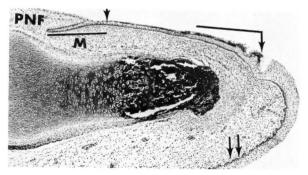

Fig. 16. Longitudinal section of 13-week-old embryo finger showing further differentiation of nail field. PNF is already formed by matrix primordium, or future matrix (M). Short arrow down indicates earliest lunula and site of earliest nail plate. Bent arrow down shows distal ridge demonstrating keratinization process much like stratum corneum of plantar-palmar epidermis. Double arrow down shows development of epidermal rete or eccrine gland alange. Phalanx now calcified. H&E X80.[1]

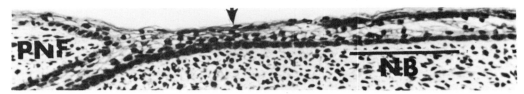

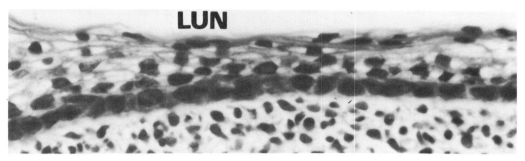

Fig. 17. High power of line above matrix (M) in Fig. 16, showing area of lunula (arrow down) where first sign of nail plate formation is seen. PNF can be seen, as well as nail bed (NB). H&E X260.

Fig. 18. Higher magnification of area of lunula (LUN) demonstrating future nucleated nail plate cells. H&E X420.

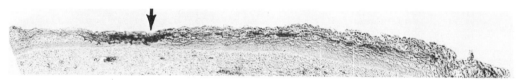

Fig. 19. Area of lunula (short arrow down) in Fig 5. 16, 17 and 18, showing strongly positive sulfhydryl stain in area of earliest nail plate formation. Barnett and Seligman stain, X98.[1]

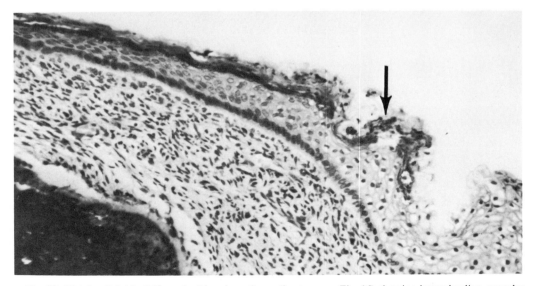

Fig. 20. Distal nail field of 13-week-old embryo finger (bent arrow, Fig. 16) showing keratohyaline granular layer as part of differentiating process of nail field epidermis. H&E X260.

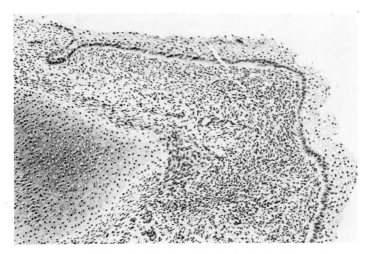

Fig. 21. Toe of 13-week-old embryo showing lag in development compared to similar aged fingernail in Fig. 16. H&E X80.

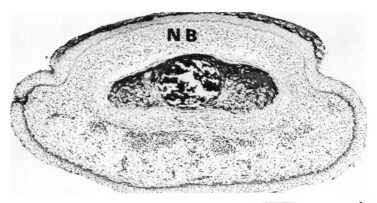

Fig. 22. Cross-section of finger in Fig. 16 at level of nail bed (NB), showing epidermal rete forming and presence of cornified layer of skin. H&E X80.

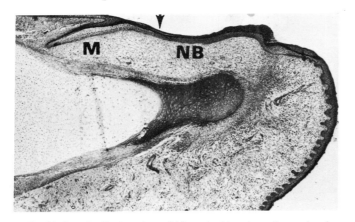

Fig. 23. Longitudinal section of 14-week-old embryo finger showing matrix primordium now producing matrix cells and r 𝑎 ' plate. Arrow down points to formed nail plate. Epidermal rete of volar plantar skin is present, with small anlage of sweat gland now visible. H&E X50.[1]

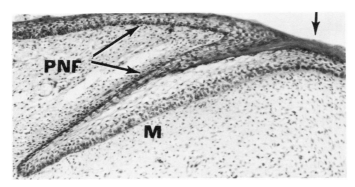

Fig. 24. Enlargement of matrix area of finger in Fig. 23, showing matrix (M) and earliest recognizable vacuolated nail plate (NP) cells. PNF is labeled for structure identification. H&E X120.[1]

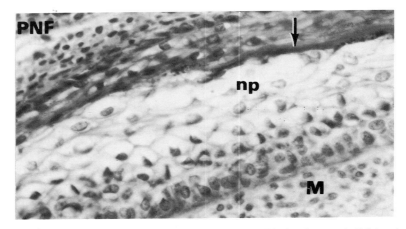

Fig. 25. Higher magnification of matrix area in Fig. 24, showing matrix (M) basal cells undergoing earliest recognizable differentiation to nail plate cells (NP), which are seen as vacuolated. H&E X460.[1]

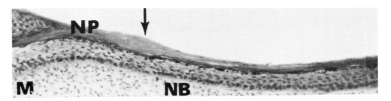

Fig. 26. Close-up of area distal to that in Fig. 24 (arrow down), showing junction between new nail plate (NP) and horny layer of nail bed (NB), which exhibits granular zone. H&E X120.

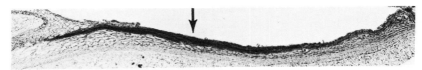

Fig. 27. Sulfhydryl stain of area in Fig. 26, showing that nail plate (NP) is quite developed but fails in H&E stain to be completely transparent at this early stage. Stratum corneum of proximal nail fold (PNF) does not stain. Barnett and Seligman stain, X120.[1]

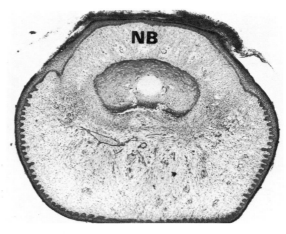

Fig. 28. Cross-section of 14-week-old embryo finger at level of nail bed (NB) showing fully developed differentiated nail bed epithelium with granular zone. H&E X50.

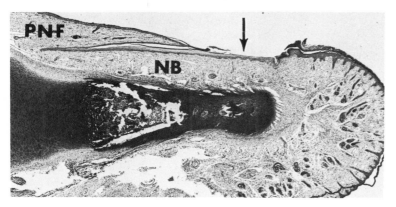

Fig. 29. Longitudinal finger of 17-week-old embryo showing proximal nail fold (PNF), nail bed (NB) and nail plate (NP) moving distally (arrow down). Epidermal rete and sweat glands are already developed in dermis of volar epithelium. H&E X28.[1]

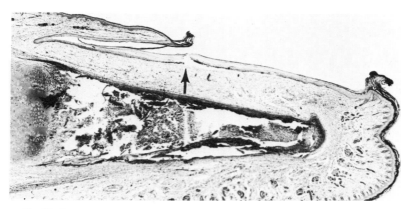

Fig. 30. Twenty-week-old finger showing notched lunula (arrow up). In gross specimen, nail plate (NP) has reached distal edge. Further development of sweat gland is seen. H&E X25.[1]

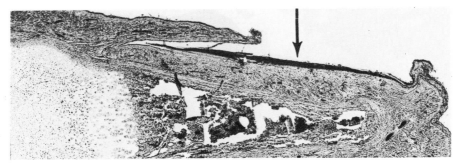

Fig. 31. Twenty-week-old finger stained with sulfhydryl stains to show massive nail plate (arrow down). Barnett and Seligman stain, X25.

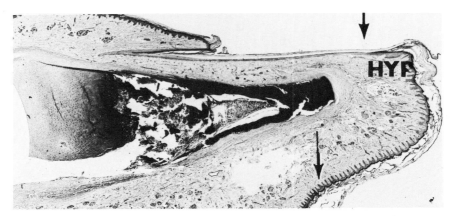

Fig. 32. Thirty-two-week-old finger showing that nail plate (short arrow down) is now past distal ridge, creating hyponychium (HYP). Large arrow down indicates well-formed epidermal rete. H&E X13.[1]

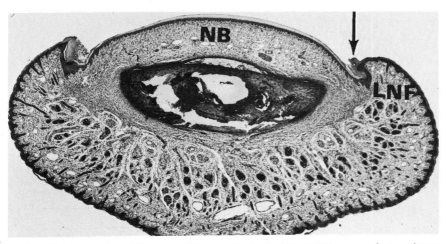

Fig. 33. Cross-section of 17-week-old finger at level of nail bed (NB). Arrow down points to lateral nail fold (NF) cuticle. Well-formed eccrine sweat glands fill volar aspects of fingertip. H&E X28.[1]

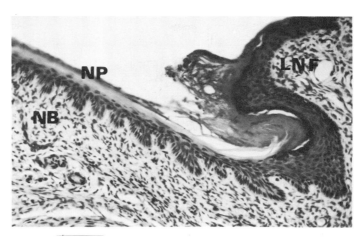

Fig. 34. Higher magnification of fig. 33, showing nail plate arrangement at lateral nail fold. Nail bed shows interlacing epidermal and dermal ridges. H&E X120.[1]

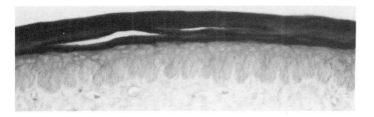

Fig. 35. Sulfhydryl-stained nail plate at level of nail bed in Fig. 34, showing positive reaction. Barnett and Seligman stain, X200.[1]

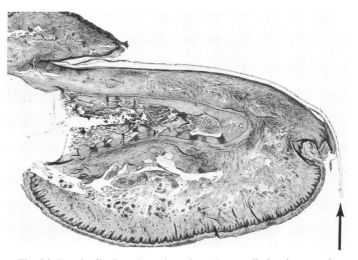

Fig. 36. Longitudinal section of newborn fingernail showing very long nail plate (arrow up) which is easily torn by cleansing of newborn. Finger structures at this stage are as in adult but smaller in size. H&E X10.[1]

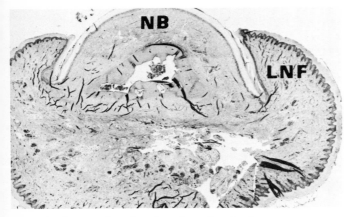

Fig. 37. Cross-section of newborn fingertip at level of nail bed showing deeply set nail plate in lateral nail fold. H&E X16.

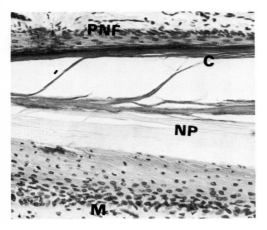

Fig. 38. Higher magnification of relationships at proximal nail fold and keratogenous zone of matrix at newborn stage. Note that cuticle is stratum corneum of nail fold and nail plate is horny end product of matrix. H&E X230.

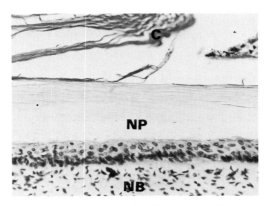

Fig. 39. Higher power of newborn fingernail at level of nail bed showing nail bed epithelium being overridden by nail plate. Cuticle of proximal nailfold at this point overrides nail plate (NP). H&E X230.[1]

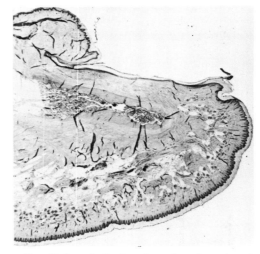

Fig. 40. Longitudinal section of newborn toe of same embryo showing lag in development of structures. H&E X10.

NOTES

1. Zaias, N.: Embryology of the human nail. *Arch. Derm. 87*: 37-53, 1963.

CHAPTER 3

Regeneration

How the nail unit regenerates or repairs itself is of great practical importance. The contribution of each nail component toward the reconstruction of the intact nail unit after trauma must be known so that in planned surgery or accidental trauma the surgeon will be aware of the repair process. Since anatomically the primate nail unit is almost identical to that of humans (Figs. 1, 2), a summary of events demonstrating how the nail unit regenerates itself is presented below.

The forcible avulsion of the nail plate denudes the surface of the digit epithelium (Fig. 3) except for the matrix (arrows). From the lateral fold and hyponychial epithelium, newly formed basaloid cells migrate and attempt to cover the denuded nail bed area (Figs. 4, 5). The matrix does not contribute to the repair of the defect (Fig. 7). A crust consisting of remaining inflammatory and necrotic epithelium cells covers the surface of the digit (Fig. 6). At first, the reepithelialized nail bed is acanthotic (Fig. 8) and exhibits a granular zone much the same as in its early developmental stages. However, as time passes, the acanthosis of the nail bed decreases. Its differentiation process reverts to one with no granular layer (Fig. 9). This is coordinated with the growth of the newly formed nail plate (Fig. 9). The process takes 18 days to complete.

Damage to the nail bed does not result in dystrophy of the nail plate. Nevertheless, the surgeon must reconstruct the nail bed in such a way as to avoid a pulling away from the future overriding nail plate.

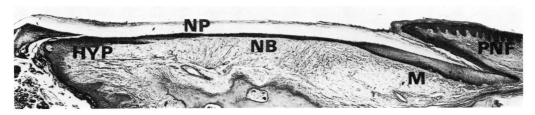

Fig. 1. Longitudinal section of primate nail prior to avulsion. *Note:* All nail unit structures are similar to human. H&E X12'

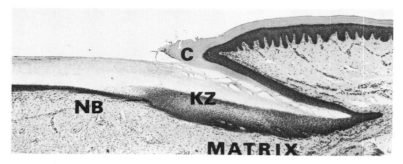

Fig. 2. Close-up of proximal nail fold (PNF) with horny cuticle (C). Matrix (M) with keratogenous zone (KZ) produces nail plate (NP). Nail bed (NB) is similar to human. H&E X50.[1]

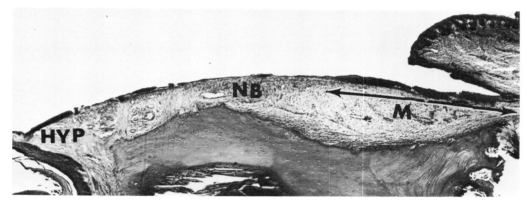

Fig. 3. Fifteen minutes after forcible avulsion of nail plate. Matrix remains intact (arrow) while epithelium of nail bed (NB) and hyponychium (HYP) are denuded. H&E X20.[1]

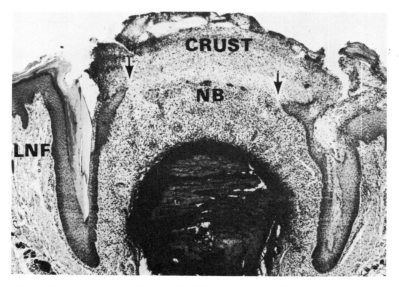

Fig. 4. Cross-section of digit at nail bed 24 hours after avulsion. From lateral nail fold epithelium, basaloid cells migrate medially (arrows) to cover defect, which is termporarily encrusted. H&E X50.[1]

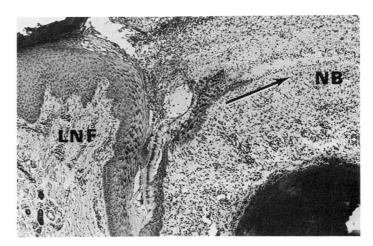

Fig. 5. High power of LNF area in Fig. 4, showing lateral nail fold epithelium "stretching" over denuded area of surface of digit (arrow), attempting to reform nail bed (NB). H&E X60.[1]

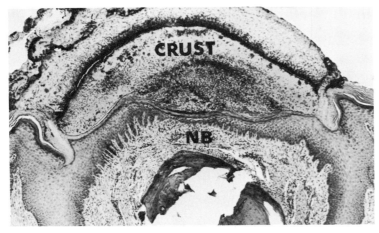

Fig. 6. Cross-section of fingertip 4 days after avulsion of nail plate at level of nail bed, showing once-denuded dorsum of finger epithelium defect. H&E X20.[1]

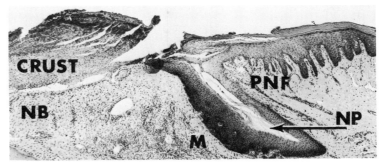

Fig. 7. Longitudinal section of finger 48 hours after avulsion. Matrix is forming nail plate and is not contributing to dorsum of finger epithelium defect. H&E X20.[1]

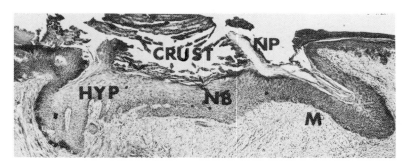

Fig. 8. Longitudinal section of digit 6 days after avulsion, showing acanthotic nail bed (NB) and matrix (M). Nail plate is overriding crust. H&E X20.

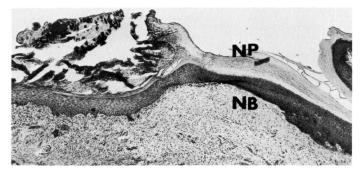

Fig. 9. Longitudinal section of finger 7 days after avulsion, showing decrease of acanthosis of nail bed (NB). H&E X50.[1]

NOTES

1. Zaias, N.: Regeneration of the primate nail: studies of the squirrel monkey, Saimiri. *J. Inv. Derm.* *44:* 107-117, 1964.

CHAPTER 4

Kinetics

Each of the four constituents of the nail unit has its own characteristic epithelial kinetics. The matrix, producing the nail plate, and the nail bed, producing horn cells which adhere to the nail plate's underside, move at the same rate and thus keep the architectural relationship of the nail plate/nail bed as a unit. The nail matrix with its nail plate is analogous to the hair matrix with its hair cortex; the nail bed and its horny layer is analogous to the inner hair root sheath. Nail bed basal cells migrate the length of the bed and differentiate all its length in virtually the same manner as the inner hair root sheath basal cells. The hyponychium (its counterpart in hair is the outer root sheath) and the proximal nail fold are like the skins to which they are respectively adjacent.

From squirrel monkey[1] and human toe studies,[2] it can be summarized that the nail plate is the horny end product of *one* epithelial germinative cell population, the matrix.

Previous theories suggesting that the nail plate is formed from three distinct matrices were based, in the opinion of this writer, on histochemical artefactual results. Moreover, nomenclature differences for similar anatomic structures compounded the lack of clarity in describing the anatomy. These theories are outlined in Table I mainly for historical purposes.

A pictorial summary of events of the movement of all nail unit components is presented at the end of this chapter. The photomicrographs show the course of radiolabeled nuclei or cytoplasm of the basal cells and the course these cells take as they become corneocytes of each nail unit component.

THE PROXIMAL NAIL FOLD (PNF) AND HYPONYCHIUM (HYP)

The PNF basal cell behaves similarly to the basal cell of the glabrous skin elsewhere. These cells, in this case labeled with tritiated glycine, move from the Malphighian layer perpendicularly to the surface to become corneocytes. The horny layer of the superficial PNF desquamates to the environment. The deeper PNF horny layer, known as the cut-

Table I

1 vs. 3 Matrices Resulting in 1 vs. 3 Nail Plate Portions

German histologists (late 1800)[3,4,5]	1	Hematoxylin-eosin stain	Human fetus
Port (early 1933)[6]	3	Polarized light studies	Human finger
Lewis (1954)[7]	3	Silver stain	Fetal finger
Achten (1963)[8]	3	Fungal penetration	Human toe
Jarrett and Spearman (1966)[9]	3	Histochemistry	Human toe
Zaias (1968)[1]	1	Glycine 3H autoradiograpgy	Monkey toe and finger
Norton (1971)[2]	1	Glycine 3H autoradiography	Human toe

icle, becomes adherent to the surface of the newly formed nail plate immediately ventral to it. The cuticle desquamates from the surface of the nail plate shortly after its emergence from under the PNF (Figs. 1, 2, 3, 4, 5). A similar sequence of events is seen in the hyponychial area. The HYP horn cells desquamate to the environment ventral to the distal free edge of the nail plate. In the HYP area covered by the nail plate, the horn cells are trapped and adhere to the ventral surface of the nail plate until they are freed from any attachment as the nail plate becomes a free edge and is then shed (Fig. 6).

THE MATRIX–NAIL PLATE

The tissue kinetics of the matrix–nail plate can be best visualized with a cytoplasmic marker, e.g., tritiated glycine or cyctine, since nuclear labels will be broken up in the upper zones of the matrix epithelium just prior to the formation of onychocytes. Again, a singly given radiolabel dose is made accessible to the basal cell and the radioactivity concentrated in the cytoplasmic proteins follows the cell's predetermined course in becoming nail plate cells.

These observations are made from monkey and rat fingers amputated at varying times after initial introduction of the radiolabel. The production of onychocytes along the entire length of the matrix occurs immediately, but it is best observed 3 days later (Fig. 7). The matrix forms a sheet of onychocytes (nail plate) along its entire length from the most proximal portion to the most distal (lunula). These cells are directed "diagonally" and distally. With further additions (growth), they extend beneath the proximal nail fold and emerge on the surface of the digit to be seen as the nail plate. Six days after the introduction of the marker, a strong black band of silver grains is seen the entire length of the matrix (Fig. 8). After 12 days, the marker is seen a third the length of the nail plate (Fig. 9); 18 days later, the marker is at the midway point. (Fig. 10). It can be summarized that:

1. The matrix is solely responsible for the formation of the nail plate.

2. The nail plate is not formed perpendicularly by the matrix and redirected by the overlying PNF, but is genetically directed diagonally and distally.

3. Portions of the matrix which are proximal form the most superficial portions and the distal matrix (lunula) form the deepest or most ventral portions of the nail plate (Fig. 1).

4. The nail plate formed by the lunula (distal matrix) is "ahead", that is, more distal than the superficial nail plate areas formed by the proximal matrix area. This supports LeGros-Clark's theory that the shape of the nail plate is related to the shape of the lunula.

5. The thickness of the nail plate is directly related to the length (size) of the matrix.

By these methods and the results obtained, the tripartite theory of nail plate formation remains unconfirmed and is hopefully as dead as the nail.

THE NAIL BED

Nuclear DNA-labeling in the nail bed basal cells suggests that the germinative cell population is situated immediately distal to the lunula, the most distal matrix area (figs. 11–16). The movement of heavily laden radiolabeled nail bed basal cells can be traced, distally, the length of the nail bed. From observations in monkey and rat nail beds, it can be concluded that:

1. Basal cells originally labeled at the nail bed origin move distally and differentiate to the surface at appropriate sites along the entire length of the nail bed. At 1 hour post-pulsing with tritiated thymidine, very heavy nuclear labeling is seen only at the germinative origin of the nail bed distal to the lunula (Fig. 2), and none is seen distally in any basal cell throughout the length of the nail bed. As time passes, likewise heavily labeled nuclei of basal cells are seen "entering" the previously unlabeled basal layer of the nail bed immediately adjacent to the originally heavily labeled germinal population (Figs. 12–16). The time required to transverse the length of the nail bed and reach the most distal nail bed adjacent to the hyponychium is as long as 18 days in squirrel monkeys and 15 days in rats.

2. The differentiation process of the nail bed from basal cells tends to occur at pre-arranged points in the basal cell area of the nail bed. The evidence for this is seen in the figures and is based on the lightening of nuclear labeling as the basal cells divide and initiate a surface movement to interlace with the lowermost onychocytes of the nail plate (Fig. 15; arrows down, Fig. 16).

3. The growth rate or movement of the matrix and nail bed cells is identical (Fig. 17), showing a band of cystine 3H label in the nail plate 3 days prior to a nuclear label to the nail bed. Both labels move in a distal jointly direction (Figs. 18, 19). A summary of the epithelial kinetics is presented in Fig. 20.

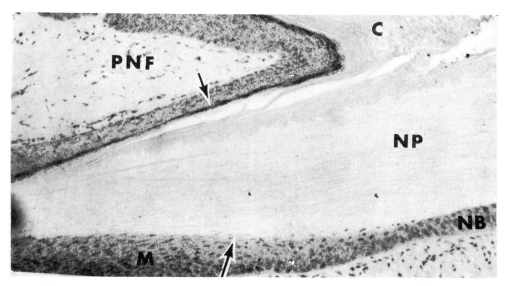

Fig. 1. Longitudinal section finger autoradiography 24 hours after dose with glycine 3H. Arrow down shows glycine incorporation into full thickness of proximal nail fold (PNF) epithelium and lowermost stratum corneum. Cuticle (C) stains differentially from nail plate (NP). Matrix (M), nail bed (NB). H&E X170.

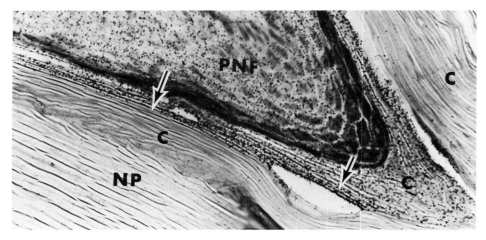

Fig. 2. PNF area 3 days post-dosing with glycine 3H. Autoradiograph showing labeled stratum corneum replacing cuticle (C) (arrow down). Nail plate (NP). H&E X450.

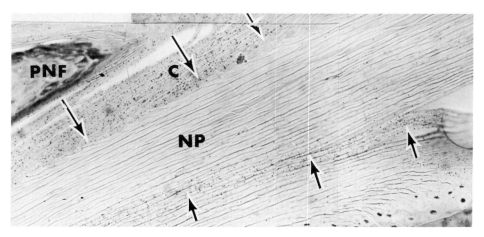

Fig. 3. PNF area 6 days post-dosing with glycine 3H. Autoradiograph showing total labeling of cuticle (C) (arrows down). Note cuticle distally is not yet labeled. Cuticle does not contribute to nail plate (NP) (arrows up). H&E X450.

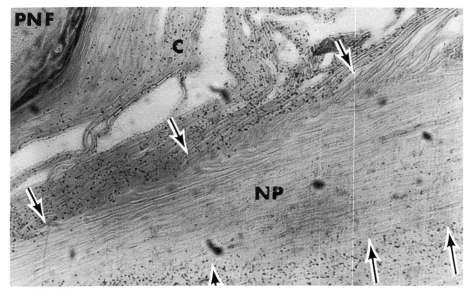

Fig. 4. PNF area 10 days post-dosing with glycine 3H. Autoradiograph showing labeled cuticle (C) (arrows up) accumulating on surface of nail plate (NP) (arrows down). PNF does not contribute to the nail plate. H&E X450.

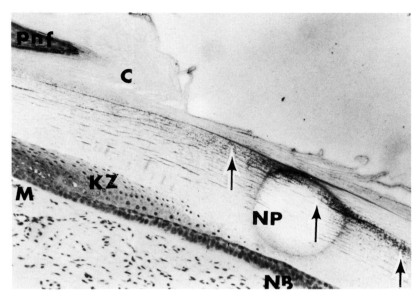

Fig. 5. PNF-lunula area 14 days post-dosing with glycine 3H. Autoradiograph showing that all of the labeled cuticle (C) has left PNF. Labeled nail plate has now emerged (arrows up) from under PNF. Keratogenous zone (KZ), Matrix (M), Nail Bed (NB). H&E X170.

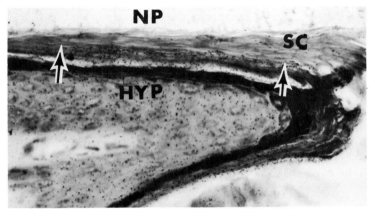

Fig. 6. Hyponychium area, longitudinal section finger 3 days post-dosing with glycine 3H autoradiograph. HYP stratum corneum can be easily differentiated (arrows up) from NP; no contribution is made to NP. H&E X470.[1]

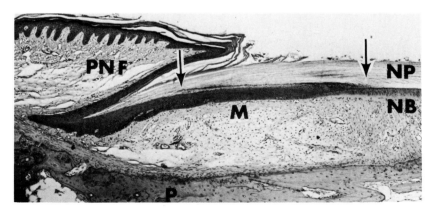

Fig. 7. Nail unit proximally, longitudinal section 3 days post–cystine 3H autoradiograph. Note black linear deposit along entire matrix (M) from PNF to NB. New nail formation (arrow down). Phalanx (P). H&E X50.

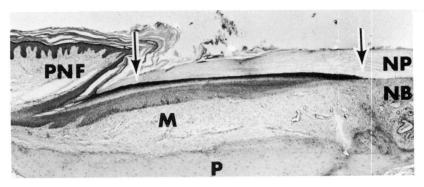

Fig. 8. Section in Fig. 7, 6 days later. Labeled NP (arrows down) clearly shows formation as one unit directed diagonally out. Proximal matrix forms superficial NP. Distal matrix forms deeper NP. H&E X50.

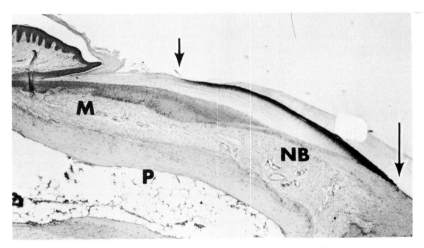

Fig. 9. Section is Figs. 7 and 8, 12 days later. Labeled NP (arrows down) substantiates legend of Fig. 8. Also it shows that thickness of NP is function of length size of Matrix H&E X76.

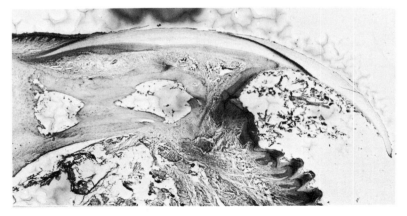

Fig. 10. Section in Figs. 7, 8 and 9, 16 days later. Labeled ventral surface NP reaches HYP area before corresponding superficial surface. Important in considering Griseofulvin therapy in onychomycosis. H&E X18.

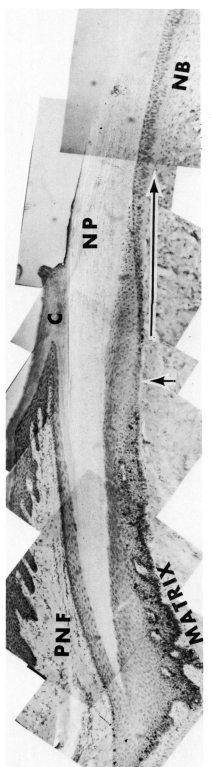

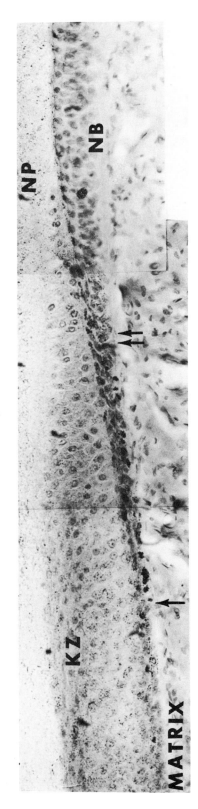

Fig. 11. Monkey finger autoradiograph 45 minutes after 3H thymidine dose. Numerous heavily labeled nuclei of matrix basal cell layer (arrows down). Similarly, heavy nuclear labeling of nail bed germinal cell epithelium (long arrow). No labeling between matrix and nail bed germinal area (arrow up). No labels distally in nail bed cells. H&E X80.

Fig. 12. High power of long-arrow area of Fig. 11. Shows nail bed germinal cell layer between single arrow up and double arrows. H&E X200.

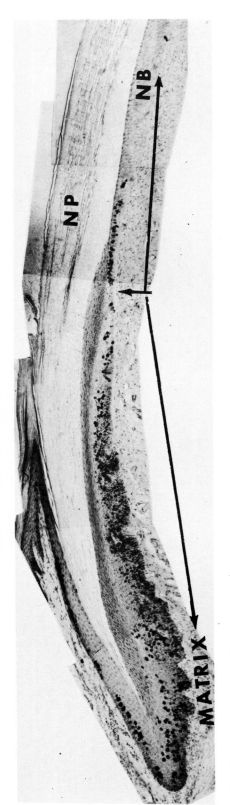

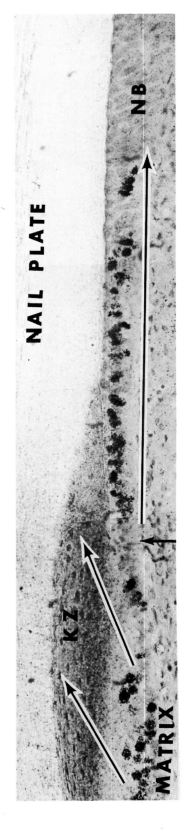

Fig. 13. Monkey finger autoradiograph 4 days post-dosing with 3H thymidine. Matrix and nail bed germinal cell population can be readily seen moving in corresponding directions; matrix diagonally out, nail bed horizontally out. Arrow up demarcates matrix from nail bed. H&E X80.

Fig. 14. High magnification of nail bed germinal cell population in Fig. 13. H&E X300.

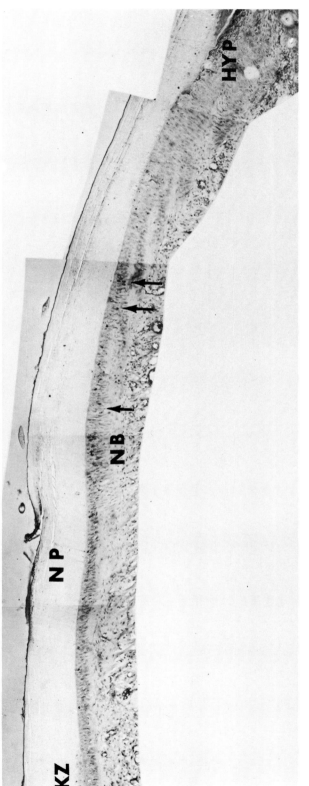

Fig. 15. Monkey finger autoradiograph 12 days post-dosing with 3H thymidine. Heavily nuclear lables are now seen midway in nail bed (arrows up). H&E X50.

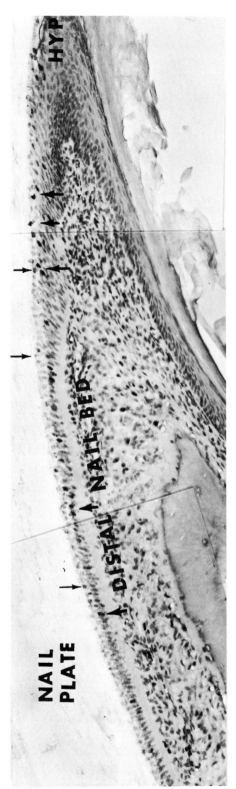

Fig. 16. Rat finger longitudinal autoradiograph 18 days post-dosing with tritiated thymidine. Heavily labeled nuclei are seen in distal areas of nail bed (arrows up). Some lighter labeled nuclei are seen differentiating as corneocytes at various points in nail bed. H&E X120.

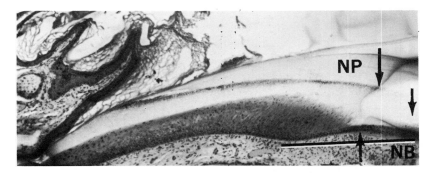

Fig. 17. Rat finger autoradiograph, double radiolabel 3 days apart. Tritiated cystine (arrows up) followed by tritiated thymidine (arrows down). H&E X120.

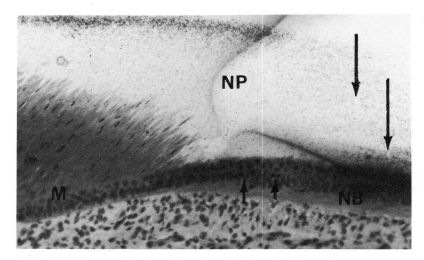

Fig. 18. Higher magnification of lunula–nail bed area in Fig. 17 (line), showing cystine label nail plate (arrows down) and nuclear labels in nail bed cells (arrows up). H&E X320.

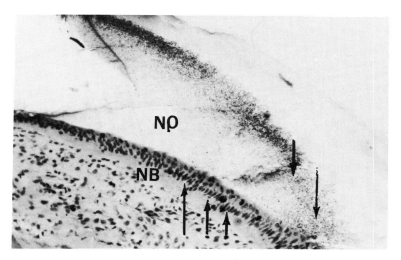

Fig. 19. Finger in Fig. 17, 7 days later, showing labeled nail plate (NP) now at mid–nail bed (arrow down) moving distally at same rate as labeled nail bed cells. H&E X320.

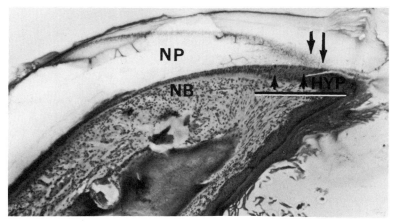

Fig. 20. Finger in Fig. 17, 14 days later, double label cystine/thymidine. Labeled nail plate (arrows down) and labeled nail bed cells (arrows up) are in same relationship (moving at same rate) and are now nearing tip of finger (hyponychium). H&E X120.

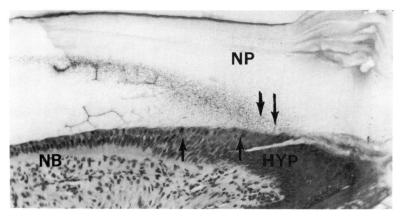

Fig. 21. Higher magnification of line in Fig. 20, clearly showing both labeled NP (arrows down) and labeled NB cells (arrows up) moving at same rate. H&E X320.

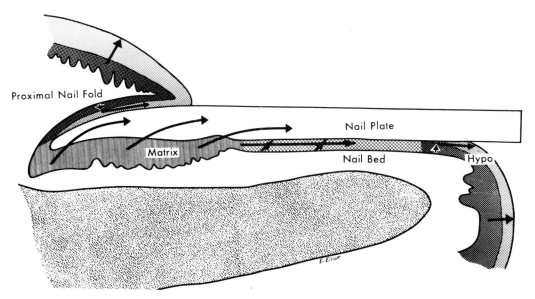

Fig. 22. Diagrammatic drawing shows direction of differentiation for proximal nail fold (PNF), matrix (M), nail bed (NB) and hyponychium (HYP).

NOTES

1. Zaias, N., and Alvarez, J.: The formation of the primate nail plate. An autoradiographic study in squirrel monkeys. *J. Invest. Derm. 51*: 120-136, 1968.
2. Norton, L.A.: Incorporation of thymidine-methyl-³H and glycine-2³H in the nail matrix and bed of humans. *J. Invest. Derm. 56*: 61-68, 1971.
3. Heynold, H.: Beitrag zur Histologie und Genese des Nagels. *Virchow Arch. Path. Anat. 65*: 270-272, 1875.
4. Zander, R.: Untersuchungen uber den Verhornungsprogress I. Die Histogenese des Nagels beim menschlichen Fetus. *Arch. Anat. Entwick 1*: 273, 1886.
5. Pollitzer, S.: Uber die Natur der won Zander im embroyonalen Nagel geiundenen Kortesrellen *Mh. Prakt. Derm. 8*: 346, 1889.
6. Port, E.: Das Auftraten von drei schichten in Derhotnsubtenz des Nagels beim der bretrechtring im Polarisierten lichte und ihre Beziehung Zur Naglematrix. *Zeitschr. Zeilforsch. Anat. 19*: 110, 1933.
7. Lewis, B.L.: Microscopic studies of fetal and mature nail and surrounding soft tissues, *Arch. Derm. Syph. 70*: 732, 1954.
8. Achten, P.G.: L'ongle normal et pathologique. *Dermatologica 126*: 229-245, 1963.
9. Jarrett, A., and Spearman, R.I.C.: The histochemistry of the human nail. *Arch. Derm. 94*: Nov. 1966.

CHAPTER 5

Hereditary And Congenital States Associated With Nail Changes

From the nail standpoint, hereditary and congenital nail changes should be categorized. An initial impression should be made of the nail unit, which may be either *overall* normal- or abnormal-looking. By and large, either matrix or nail bed abnormalities are most common. If the nail unit looks *overall* normal but there is a question as to shape and size, then a *nail bed abnormality* is indicated which may be associated with a phalangeal abnormality. If the nail unit looks abnormal, in that the nail plate is defective, hypoplastic or hypertrophic, then the defect is usually of the nail matrix.

The normal appearance of the nail unit is presented in Figs. 1, 4 and 10.

SYNDROMES WITH OVERALL NORMAL-LOOKING NAIL UNITS (Table I)

Normal nail unit with unusual pigmentation
  A. Melanin deposits—Peutz-Jeghers syndrome[1,2]
  B. Leukonychia
    1. Leukonychia associated with spoon nails and deafness; dominant knuckle pads, leukonychia and hearing loss[72]
    2. Total leukonychia[78]
    3. Partial leukonychia[76]
    4. Striated leukonychia[77]
    5. Leukonychia and koilonychia[75] (Figs. 19, 20)
    6. Leukonychia totalis, multiple sebaceous cysts and renal calculi[74]
Nail Plate appearing shorter than normal (short nail plate and/or distal phalanx) (Figures 9, 11)
  A. Associated with multiple joint dislocations, flat facies. Larsen's syndrome[7]

B. Associated with sparse fine hair, mild bowing of legs, shortened length of bones. Cartilage-hair hypoplasia[8]

Nail plate appearing broader and shorter than normal (nail bed broader and shorter) (Figs. 3, 13)

A. Associated with various system abnormalities, e.g., acrocephaly, polydactyly of feet with syndactyly, mental retardation and definitively obese. Carpenter's syndrome[13]

B. Associated with postnatal onset of thickened joint contractures, especially hands (joint limitations). Leri's pleonosteosis[14]

C. Associated with craniosynostoses (monstrous) mid-facial hypoplasia, flat facies, syndactyly and fusion. Apert's syndrome[15]

D. Associated with short stature hypoplastic maxilla, palpebral fissures slanting downwards. Rubinstein-Taybi syndrome[16,17] (possibly thin), with tapering or deepslated (overlapping lateral nail folds) (Figs. 2, 5, 8)

Nail plate appearing narrower than normal

A. Long arm 18 deletion syndrome[5]—mid-facial hypoplasia, prominant antihelix, whorl digital pattern (Fig. 2)

B. Associated with shortened or "webbed" neck female, short stature, broad chest with widespread nipples. XO syndrome (Turner's).[9] Edema of acral parts.

C. Associated with sparse fine hair, cone-shaped epipyses, pear-shaped nose, short stature. Tricho-rhino-phalangeal syndrome[65]

Nail plate exaggeratedly larger than normal (large hands and feet) (Figs. 3,6)

A. Cerebral gigantism[3] (Soto's syndrome). Large-size infant, large hands and feet; poor coordination (Figs. 3, 6)

B. Unilateral hypertrophy. Congenital hemihypertrophy syndrome[66]

Nail plate curvature abnormalities—pseudo-Clubbing (Fig. 13)

A. Associated with shortened or "webbed" neck, female, short stature, congenital lymphedema, broad chest with widespread nipples. XO syndrome (Turner's).[9] Nails not really narrowed or thin but deeply set in lateral nail fold. Edematous lateral nail fold extension over lateral aspects of nail plate gives false narrow and deepset appearance. (Figs. 2, 8)

B. Associated with polydactyly, defects of eye, nose and lips; capillary hemagioma forehead, cardiac defects, central nervous system defects of 13 Trisomy syndrome[10,11]

C. Associated with delayed eruption and teeth skeletal defects (clavicle). Cleidocranial dysostosis[12]

D. Associated with arachnodactyly, disproportionate skeletal growth, great bessels, eye and skeletal abnormalities. Marfan's syndrome[67]

E. Associated with sclerosing acral poikilodermatous skin. Hereditary sclerosing poikiloderma[68]

F. Familial koilonychia.[69] Nail plate appears flatter than normal.

G. Leukonychia and koilonychia[75]

H. Pyknodysostosis of Maroteaux and Lamy[6]—estosclerosis, short distal phalages, delayed closure of fontanels (Fig. 12)

Nail plate overall size smaller than normal (small hands and feet)

A. Werner's syndrome[4]—late childhood to early adult onset of cataract, thin skin with thick fibrous subcutaneous tissue, gray hair (Figs. 4, 10)

Abnormalities of distal groove and hyponychium (absence of distal groove, extended painful hyponychium)

A. Congenital, painful aberrant hyponychium[84] (Fig. 20; Ch. 1)

HEREDITARY AND CONGENITAL SYNDROMES WITH UNDERDEVELOPED, PLASTIC OR HYPOPLASTIC NAIL UNITS (Table II)

Nail unit changes reflecting a grossly abnormal nail plate, usually a matrix defect
  A. Focal absence of matrix/nail plate (Fig. 7)
  B. Total absence of matrix/nail plate (Fig. 14)
  C. Decreased length of matrix as compared to normal (Fig. 12); thinned nail plate

HEREDITARY AND CONGENITAL SYNDROMES WITH ABNORMAL-LOOKING AND HYPERPLASTIC NAIL UNITS

  A. Nail bed hypertrophy (Fig. 15)
    1. Hereditary hyperkeratosis of nail beds[79]
    2. Symmetrical hyperkeratosis of nail beds and palms and soles[80]
    3. Pachyonychia congenita[81,83] (Jadassohn and Lewandowsky) (Figs. 23, 24)
    4. Mental retardation, unusual facies and abnormal nails associated with a Group G-ring chromosome[82]
    5. Hereditary dystrophy of hair and nails[83]

Epidermolysis Bullosa

This congenital skin and nail disease is characterized by the formation of blisters on pressure areas of the skin. There are various clinical types with different inheritance patterns and different anatomical locations for the abnormality, which results in blisters (see Table IV and Figs. 1–3).

Bart[1] has described a child with a localized absence of skin as well as blistering of the mucosa and skin and nail dystrophy resembling epidermolysis bullosa.

Nail-Patella Syndrome—Hereditary Osteo-Onychodysplasia (Hood)

This syndrome, first described by Little[89] in 1897 because of nail changes, represents an autosomal dominant, congenital connective tissue disorder which also displays nail and skin abnormalities, probably secondary to their supporting stroma. Abnormalities generally seen are:
1. Congenital nail dystrophy
2. Absent or hypoplastic patella
3. Radial head abnormalities
4. Iliac crests (exostosis) commonly referred to as "horns"
5. Kidney (glomenular) abnormalities
Abnormalities less frequently seen are:
1. Other skeletal abnormalities, e.g., joint hyperextensibility, thickened or hypoplastic scapulae, talipes, cervical spina bifida, cervical ribs, pigeon chest, thoracic kyphosis, hyperostosis frontalis, exostosis of inner table of frontal bone, lordosis, spondylosis, scoliosis, calcaneo valgus, absent anterior cruciate ligament, clinodactyly, horizontal sacrum equinovarus, and coxa valga
2. Other skin abnormalities, e.g., webbing of popliteal areas, finger webs, absent skin creases on distal fingers

3. Eye—heterochromia of iris, cloverleaf deformities, iris cataracts, ptosis, paralysis of internal rectus

Nail Abnormalities

Lucas and Opitz[90] have reviewed the literature. Although abnormalities involving the nail are generally present at birth, two separate reports describe postnatal nail changes. Fingers are usually affected; toes rarely. Thumbs are usually affected, with index fingers next. There is a lesser incidence in remaining fingers, with 5th fingers least affected.

Nail unit changes range from total absence of nail plate (matrix absence) to damage of partial area of nail plate such as medially (medial matrix damage), thinning of nail plate (shortened matrix), narrowness of nail plate (smaller area of matrix), smallness of nail plate (smaller matrix), ridging of nail plate (damage to proximal matrix), spooning (nail bed abnormalities), softness of nail plate (very short and small matrix), median groove to nail plate (split matrix) and abnormalities of lunula from absence to abnormal shapes, e.g., triangular (Figs. 1–6).

Elbow Abnormalities

Limitation of motions (extension, pronation and supination). Subluxation of radial heads.

Kidney Abnormalities

Recent awareness of nephropathology and its serious implications has moved this syndrome from a curiosity to a serious disease. Not unusually, protenuria and hematuria are noted very early on, with persistence and often fatal outcome. At least one report describes a spontaneous improvement of kidney disease.[91] Glomerular involvement is commonplace. Electronmicroscopic studies have revealed many changes most noteworthy of which is the presence of collagen in the basement membrane.[92-94] Simila and co-workers have summarized the world literature on kidney disease and its outcome (Table V).

Acid micropolysaccharides and hydroxyproline are normal when compared to 24 hour urine levels of control. Proline, however, is significantly elevated[95] The mutation for this disease occurs near the locus for Blood ABO compatibility.

Pachyonychia Congenita

In this syndrome, primarily the nail bed becomes hyperkeratotic and elevates the nail plate. This abnormality by itself was first described by Garrick Wilson in 1905[79] as hereditary hyperkeratosis of the nail beds. Earlier, in 1897, Colcott Fox[80] described the nail changes in association with palmar and plantar keratosis. It was not until 1906 that the full syndrome was described by Jadassohn and Lewandosky.[86] This genodermatosis appears to have an autosomal dominant inheritance pattern with incomplete penetrance.

Supposedly seen more frequently among Jewish and Slavic males, this syndrome is infrequently reported. The full syndrome consists of:
1. Abnormal fingers and toenails
2. Hyperhidrosis of palms and soles
3. Mildly ichthyotic skin wih accentuated follicular papules
4. Focal and usually symmetrical palmar and plantar hyperkeratosis; bullae are frequently described during warm weather; following such bullae, deep ulcerations may result which vary in depth and may be very painful
5. Leukokeratosis on the tongue and oral mucosa
6. Verrucosities over knees, elbows, buttocks and popliteal areas
7. Corneal hyskeratosis, cataracts
8. Hoarseness, deafness
9. Presence of teeth at birth
10. Reported with short stature
11. Reported with mental retardation
12. Reported with steatocystoma multiplex
13. Reported with epidermolysis bullosa
14. Reported with oral herpetic lesions
15. Reported with elevated serum iron and copper
16. Reported with elevated excretion of hydroxy proline and hexosamine in urine

The nails are the most characteristic signs. Patients are usually born with normal nails. Shortly after 3 to 5 months, a reddish-brown nail bed discoloration is noted. This is followed by a thickening of the nail bed which eventually results in:
1. Remarkable elevation of nail plate (Fig. 30)
2. Lateral compression of nail plate (Fig. 31)

These are usually seen in fingernails. The toenails may show only marked nail bed keratosis.

The nail plates have been described as yellow, tan or brown. The nail plate may fall off, leaving a blackish pellicle. All these colors after the nail plate elevates are probably due to colonization of bacteria. The skin and mucosa, most commonly of the soles, palms, knees, elbows, popliteal, buttocks and tongue, tend to become thickened focally. The larynx (hoarseness) oral cavity, tympanic membrane (deafness) and follicular orifices tend to become plugged. Serum copper and iron have been described as elevated, as has excretion of hydroxy proline and hexosamine in 24 hour urines. Thormann and Kabaysi[96] studied one patient by electromicroscopy and concluded that the disorder was a hereditary dyskeratosis.

Histopathology

The nail bed epidermis is hyperplastic. There is acanthosis and, characteristically, a great deal of hyperkeratosis and focal parakeratosis. The keratinazation process of the nail bed is completely abnormal. Originating from the basal layer are characteristic cells of the Malpighian layer which contain an eosinophylic cytoplasm very similar to what may be called "individual cell keratinazation" (these cells are not atypical). From the Malpighian layer, such unusual keratinocytes become stratum corneum cells. These observations were made from two biopsies of the nail bed (mother and daughter). This probably represents a Dyskeratotic genodermatosis.

Table I
Hereditary and Congenital Syndromes With Overall "Normal-Looking" Nail Units

Apert
Carpenter
Cartilage-hair hypoplasia
Cleidocranial dysostosis
Congenital painful hyponychium
Curtis syndrome, hemi-gigantism
Dominant knuckle pads, leukonychia and hearing loss
Dysplasia epiphysealis multiplex
Familial koilonychia
Hereditary dystrophy of hair and nails
Hereditary sclerosing poikiloderma
Larsen
Leri's plenosteosis
Leukonychia and koilonychia (Figs. 19, 20)
Leukonychia totalis, sebaceous cysts and renal calculi
Long arm 18 deletion syndrome
Marfan
Partial leukonychia
Peutz-Jeghers
Pyknodysostosis of Maroteaux and Lamy
Raquet nails
Rubinstein-Taybi
Soto's cerebral gigantism
Striated leukonychia
Total leukonychia
13 Trisomy
Tricho-rhino-phalangeal
Unilateral hypertrophy syndrome
Werner
XO (Turner)

Table II
Hereditary and Congenital Syndromes With Underdeveloped, Absent or Hypoplastic Nail Units (Matrix-Plate)

Syndrome	Reference	Comments	Inheritance
Index fingers—congenital nonhereditary onychodysplasia (C.O.I.F.,Iso)	18,49,50	Only index fingers, occasional phalanx abnormalities, mostly reported in Japanese literature	Noninherited
Simple anonychia	20	No underlying phalanges abnormality	Autosomal recessive
Anonychia with ectrodactyly	21,51	Absence of distal phalanges	Autosomal dominant
Coffin and Siris syndrome— anonychia, ectrodactyly and mental retardation	53	Exclusively 5th finger abnormality	Not known
Hereditary onychodysplasia of 5th toenails—autosomal dominant	52	Toenail present but nail plate abnormal	Autosomal dominant

Syndrome	Reference	Comments	Inheritance
Incontinentia pigmenti (Bloch-Sulzberger)	32	Approximately 7% of reported cases worldwide have nail plate dystrophy, probably 2nd to vesicular formation of matrix	Undetermined
Ectodermal dysplasia —Basan type	23	Thin, fragile nail plates, simian creases, smooth palms and soles	Autosomal dominant
Ectodermal dysplasia— Clouston type	24	Hypoplasia to aplasia of nail plates; Hair hypoplasia to alopecia; palms and soles	Autosomal dominant
Drug-induced— Aminopterin, Hydantoin, M.O.P.P.	25,47,64	Matrix nail plate abnormalities noted	Not known
Enamel hypoplasia and curly hair	28	Nail matrix–nail plate changes may or may not occur; teeth peculiarly worn down	Autosomal dominant
Dyskeratosis congenita	26	Great variability of nail matrix–nail plate changes; skin hyperpigmentation may be since birth; pancytopenia; malignant degeneration of mucosal leukoplasia. may develop; many other systems involved	Autosomal recessive
Chondroectodermal dysplasia (Ellis–Van Creveld)	27	Nails may be hypoplastic (short stature, short extremities); hand functions may be impaired; inability to clench fist	Autosomal recessive
Ectodermal dysplasia— Feinmesser type	29	Short fissured nail plate; spooning, dystrophic congenital deafness and onychodystrophy	Autosomal recessive
Focal dermal hypoplasia (Goltz)	30	Mesoectodermal abnormalities very similar in expression to incontinentia pigmenti; usually females; skin atrophy with lipomatous protrusions; other symptoms involved.	Not Known
Ectodermal dysplasia—hypohidrotic	31	Variability in nail matrix–nail plate abnormalities (hypoplastic); decreased to no sweating, abnormal teeth, saddle nose	X-linked
Enchodromatosis (Maffucci)	33	Hematomata; enchondroma displasing matrix results in nail plate changes	Autosomal dominant
Nail-patella syndrome— Hereditary osteo-onychodysplasia (Hood) (Fig. 24)	34	Nail matrix–nail plate variability; hypoplastic changes (nail plate splitting, iliac spurs 80%, iris, renal and CNS changes); pointed lunula (triangular) commonly in thumbnail, patella absent 92%; small head radius 90%; mid-posterior in 98%	Autosomal dominant
Oculo-dento-digital	35	Aplasia of one or more distal phalanges, no nail unit; eye, nose, teeth, hands and feet rare	Autosomal dominant
Oto-palato-digital (Taybi)	36	Thumbnail abnormalities, short stature, deafness, facial bone hypoplasia. Extremities abnormalities.	Unclear
Poland's anomaly	37	Nail dystrophy, unilateral, failure of limbs to develop; pectoral musculature abnormalities	Not inherited

Syndrome	Reference	Comments	Inheritance
Popliteal web syndrome (Trelat)	38	Toenail dysplasia, proximal nail fold perimeter convex rather than concave; tendency to split nail plate into two portions; oral abnormalities (palate, lips, etc.); webbing by skin in popliteal area and others	Not Known
Progeria (Abiotrophic disease Hutchinson -Gilford)	39	Brittle, crumbly nail plate, onset in infancy; premature aging—alopecia, atrophy of subcutaneous fat, skeletal dysplasia	Autosomal recessive
Ecotodermal dysplasia—Robinson type	40	**Hypoplastic** and dystrophic nails; abnormal teeth, sensorineural hearing loss	Autosomal dominant
Poililoderma congenita (Rothmund)	41	Hypoplastic and dystrophic nails; poikilodermatous skin by 1st year of life; cataracts by 7 years; other skin and teeth problems	Autosomal recessive
Streeter's bands	42	Hypoplasia of limb or part of limb secondary to amnion strangle	Not inherited
Tuberous sclerosis (fig. 22)	43	Multiple harmartoma fibro-angiomas of skin occurring in, on and under nail matrix; so-called subungual fibroma, Shagreen patches, "adenoma sebaceous" in face, eye, brain, bone and kidney	
Chromosome 18 trisomy syndrome	44	Extraordinary variable number of abnormalities; hypoplastic finger and toenails	
Chromosome long arm 21 deletion syndrome (anti-mongolism)	45	Hypoplastic nails; down slanting palpebral fissure, ear and mouth abnormalities; very rare	Not known
Triphalangy of thumbs and great toes	46	Hypoplastic or absent nails of thumbs and great toes, associated with triphalangy; Tooth and dermatoglyphic abnormalities; deafness, convulsive disorders and mental retardation	Autosomal dominant X-linked dominant(?)
Hypohidrotic ectodermal dysplasia with multiple associated abnormalities (Rapp-Hodgkins) (Figs. 16, 17, 18)	54,55	Hypoplastic nails with anhidrotic ectodermal syndrome abnormalities and, in addition, short stature, cleft lip palate, hypospadios, eye and other abnormalities.	Autosomal dominant
Curly hair—ankyloblepharon nail dysplasia (Chands)	56	Nail hypoplasia, curly hair, ankyloblepharon, ataxia(?)	Autosomal dominant
Glossopalatine ankylosis Microglossia, hypodontia, abnormalities of extremities	48	Nails hypoplastic to absent; ankylosis of tongue to hard palate, andontia, cleft palate, abnormalities of hands and feet	Not known
Absence of phalanges and toenails	57	Absence of distal phalanges of toes 2,3,4 with anonychia	Not Known
Ectromelia—unilateral, psoriasis and central nervous system anomalies (Fig. 21)	58	Nail plate dystrophic, psoriatic; familial psoriasis	Not known

Syndrome	Reference	Comments	Inheritance
Cryptophthalmia syndrome	59	Nail matrix–nail plate hypoplastic; often shared by various syndactylous toes and fingers; eyebrows missing, skin covering eyes, small ears, bizarre hairline, bilateral cryptophalmia, eye defects; many other system abnormalities	Autosomal recessive
Chromosome Type C trisomy	60	Nail matrix–nail plate hypoplasia, shortened fingers	Not known
Keratosis palmo-plantaris associated with heliotrichia	61	Hypoplastic congenital nail plates; splitting	Not known
Sclero-atrophying and keratodermic genodermatosis of extremities	62	Hypoplastic fingernails, from streaking to anonychia—sclerodactyly, erythocyanosis, atrophic skin kerotoderma	Autosomal dominant
Impaired growth and onchodysplacia (Senior)	63	Short stature, mental retardation, impaired growth, hypoplastic toenails	Not known
Dominant onychodystrophy and hearing loss	70	Nail changes and deafness	Autosomal dominant
Recessive onychodystrophy Digital abnormalities and hearing loss	71	Low IQ, clinodactyly, camptodactyly, rudimentary nose, deafness	Autosomal recessive

Table III

Syndromes with Nail Abnormalities and Hearing Loss[73]

Dominant onychodystrophy and hearing loss[70]
Feinmesser-type ectodermal defects[29]
Knuckle pads, leukonychia and deafness[72]
Recessive onychodystrophy, digital abnormalities and deafness[71]
Robinson-type ectodermal dysplasia[40]
Taybi's syndrome (oto-palato-digital)[36]
Triphalangy of thumbs and great toes[46]

Table IV*

Classification of the Mechanobullous Diseases

Skin Involvement	Nail Involvement
NON-SCARRING	
Epidermolysis bullosa simplex	Mildly involved Usually no scarring
Recurrent bullous eruption, hands and feet (Weber-Cockayne)	No
Junctional bullous epidermatosis (epidermolysis bullosa hereditaria letallis)	May involve nail area with scarring
SCARRING	
Dermolytic bullous disease	
Dominant type (epidermolysis bullosa dystrophica hyperplastica)	Yes
Recessive type (epidermolysis bullosa dystrophica polydysplasia)	Yes
Acquired type	Mild changes

*Adapted from Pearson.[88]

Table V

Incidence of Nephropathy-Hood and Fatal Nephropathy-Hood in Families of Hood*

Family Members with Hood	Family Members with Nephropathy and Hood	Family Members with Fatal Nephropathy and Hood
173	52 (30%)	14 (26%)

*Simila et al., 1970.

Acrodermatitis Enteropathica

Acrodermatitis enteropathica (AE) is a rare familial disease (autosomal recessive) usually manifesting itself before 18 months of age. Adults have exhibited a similar syndrome, but AE is definitely a pediatric disease. Although the clinical syndrome has been well-described since 1942,[97] its cause was unknown until zinc deficiency was implicated in a variant of acrodermititis enteropathica with lactose intolerance.[98] This fact has been confirmed by other investigators who have, in addition, tried to explain how all the symptoms and signs in AE are interlaced to zinc absorption and metabolism.

Characteristically, the syndrome consists of:

1. A skin eruption involving acral and periorificial areas
2. Alopecia
3. Nail unit involvement
4. Diarrhea

Other symptoms and their incidence have been tabulated by Wells and Winkelman[99] and appear in Table VI.

Skin

The skin lesions are primarily vesiculo-bullous and tend to dry and crust, resulting in large psoriasiform sheets of scale. These areas may become impetiginous, with large amounts of exudation and erythema. Verrucosities appear in some cases, resulting in grotesque skin changes, and keratodermia of the palms and soles may be seen. Skin lesions heal without scarring or atrophy. Some investigators[100-102] have speculated that there is an essential fatty acid interconversion defect. In mild cases, serum fatty acids are of normal levels; this is probably due to the breakdown of body fat and the decrease of delivery of fat to skin rather than normal absorption through the gut. In severe cases, fat stores are depleted to such a degree that low serum fatty acid abnormalities result.

Nails

Red paronychial areas and elevation of the nail plate, secondary to nail bed epidermal hyperplasia give the appearance of an enlarged digit. Impetiginous exudation from the proximal nail fold and from under the nail plate finally results in the shedding of the nail plate, exposing the eczematous nail bed. The nail plate has been described as thickened, but careful description has not been reported.

Diarrhea

The mucosa of the small intestine in AE has been reported to be abnormally structured. Concomitant with these changes, the patient exhibits diarrhea. Zinc therapy has reversed the gastrointestinal changes with disappearance of the diarrhea.[103]

Treatment

Prior to 1953, human breast milk was considered very effective in the treatment of AE. In 1953, Schlomovitz suggested and Dillaha, Lorencz and Aavik[104] reported the successful use of diiodohydroxtquin (Diodoquin) in the treatment of AE. It was not until later, however, that Moynahan and Barnes[98] suggested and proved that AE and some of its variants are zinc state deficiencies. Presently, there is much speculation about how variably abnormal fatty acid metabolism, abnormal structure and histochemical data of the mucosa of the duodermal and small bowel, and skin lipid deposition are all correlated with zinc deficiency.

Diodoquin tablets each contain 300 micrograms of zinc. The mechanism of action of Diodoquin proposed by Delves, Harris, Lawson and Mitchell[105] simply suggests that Diodoquin binds to zinc and other metals (copper, iron and manganese), facilitating their absorption through the enterocyte. Diodoquin given with a zinc-deficient diet failed to improve one patient with AE.[107] A decreased cellular immunity has been described in AE and has been directly associated with zinc deficiency; once the deficiency was corrected, the cellular immunity became normal.[106]

A zinc deficiency state can be best determined by zinc concentrations of hair.[108]

Table VI

Frequency of Predominant Findings in 58 Reported Cases of AE[99]

	%
Skin lesions	100
Alopecia	98
Paronychia	96
Nail dystrophy	96
Diarrhea	91
Growth change	83
Familial history	65
Cutaneous or mucous membrane candidiasis	56
Mental change	41

In addition, glossitis and stomatitis, photophobia, conjunctivitis, perleche, and corneal opacities have been reported. Low zinc stores have been reported in bronchial abnormalities, beta lipoprotenemia, alpha-gamma globulemenia and fibrocystic disease.

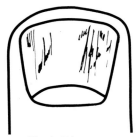

Fig. 1. Diagrammatic drawing of normal nail unit.

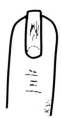

Fig. 2. Diagrammatic drawing of micronychia. Small Finger, narrow nail bed area and matrix.

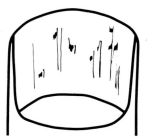

Fig. 3. Macronychia. Wider than usual nail bed and matrix.

Fig. 4. Diagrammatic drawing, cross-section of normal nail.

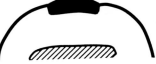

Fig. 5. Cross-section of micronychia (Fig. 2) showing reduced, narrowed nail bed width.

Fig. 6. Cross-section of Fig. 3, showing wider than usual nail bed unit.

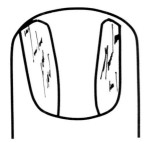

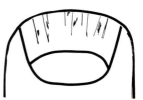

Fig. 7. Diagrammatic drawing of focal atrophy, with absence of matrix and two lateral nail plate remnants left. A common abnormality in congenital dystrophic nails.

Fig. 8. Cross-section of what appears clinically to be micronychia (Fig. 2) but is in fact overlapping of nail unit area by lateral nail folds. Described in Turner's syndrome.

Fig. 9. Nail unit with short nail bed area as compared to Figs. 1 and 3.

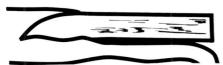

Fig. 10. Diagrammatic drawing, longitudinal appearance, of normal nail unit.

Fig. 11. Diagrammatic drawing of shortened nail bed. Nail unit appearing clinically like Fig. 9.

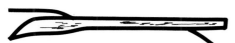

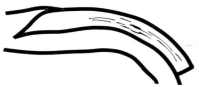

Fig. 12 Diagrammatic drawing of very thin nail plate, normal size of nail bed (shortened nail matrix results in thinner nail plate).

Fig. 13 Curved nail plate, due to curvature of digit surface not seen normally.

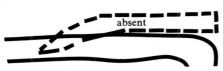

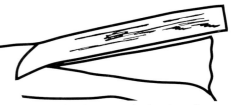

Fig. 14. Diagrammatic drawing of anonychia (absent nail plate) seen in dystrophic states.

Fig. 15. Diagrammatic drawing of hypertrophic nail unit as in pachonychia congenita, where nail bed is hypertrophied and matrix is thickened, producing thickened and elevated nail plate.

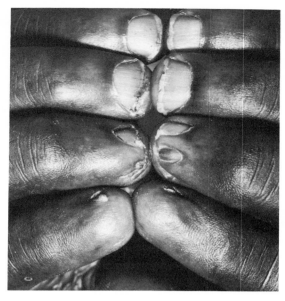

Fig. 16. Patient with congenital ectodermal defect. Note that some nails are absent and some have partial remnants of nail. (University of Miami)

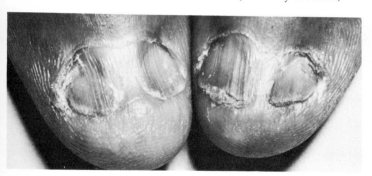

Fig. 17. Close-up of thumbs of patient in Fig. 16. (University of Miami)

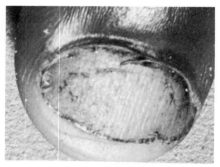

Fig. 18. Thin nails similar to those in Fig. 12, also seen in many congenital ectodermal defects. (University of Miami)

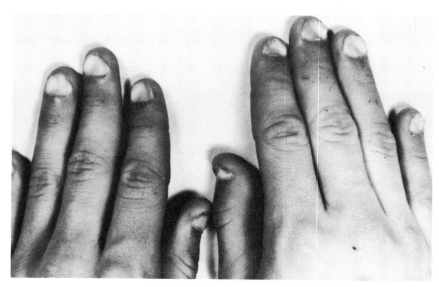

Fig. 19. White (leukonychic) koilonychia. Combination is seen in patients also having hearing deficits. See Table III.

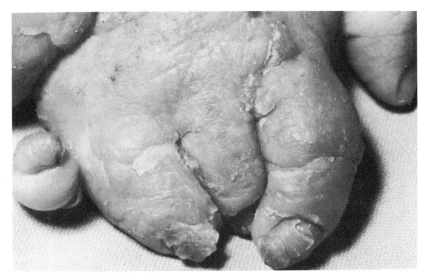

Fig. 20. Psoriasisiform changes in skin, nails and bone abnormalities in ectromelia. (Dr. Shear, University of Miami.)

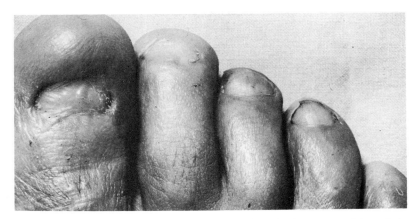

Fig. 21. Toes of patient with epidermolysis bullosa, (dominant type of dermolytic bullous disease) (epidermalyis bullosa dystophic Hyperplastica). (University of Miami)

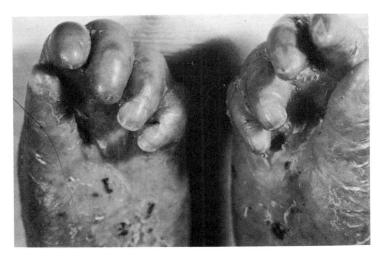

Fig. 22. Hands of patient with dermolytic bullous disease, recessive type (epidermolysis bullosa dystrophic polydysplasia), showing fusion of skin between fingers and absence of fingernails as result of blistering. (University of Miami)

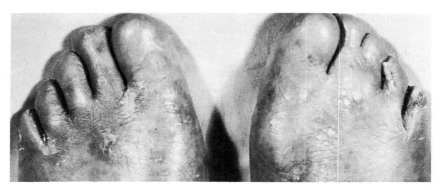

Fig. 23. Feet and toes of patient in Fig. 22. (University of Miami)

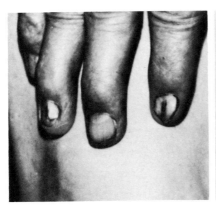

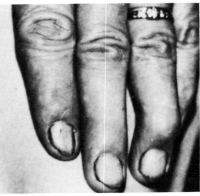

Fig. 24. Nails of patient with nail-patella syndrome. Note variation of abnormalities in index finger and ring finger.[90]

Fig. 25 Fingers of patient in Fig. 24. In addition to abnormality of index finger nail unit, note bone abnormality of ring finger.[90]

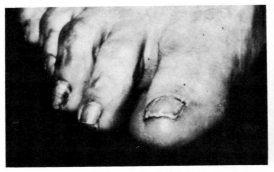

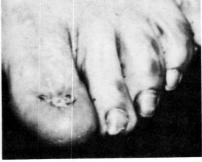

Fig. 26. Toes of patient in Fig. 24 showing bone abnormalities as well as minor nail changes.[90]

Fig. 27. Patient in Fig. 24, showing anonychia.[90]

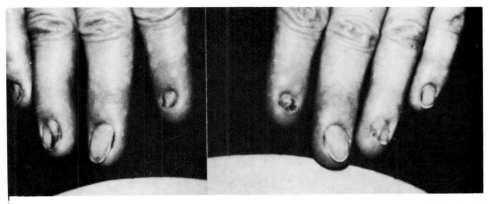

Figs. 28 and 29. Fingernails of patient in Figs. 26 and 27, showing variation and abnormalities of nail bed and matrix.[90]

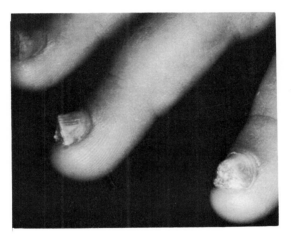

Fig. 30. Pachonychia congenita. 32-year-old female. Note hypertrophy of nail bed and lateral curvature of nail plate.

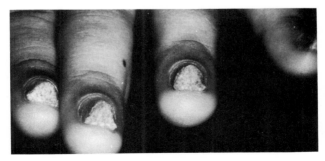

Fig. 31. Similar end view showing hypertrophy of nail bed.

NOTES

1. Jeghers, H., McKusick, V.A., and Katz, K.H.: Generalized intestinal polyposis and melanin spots of the oral mucosa, lips and digits. A syndrome of diagnostic significance. *New Eng. J. Med. 241*: 933, 1949.
2. Reid, J.D.: Intestinal carcinoma in the Peutz-Jeghers Syndrome. *JAMA 229*: 833-834, 1974.
3. Stephenson, J.N., Mellinger, R.C., and Manson, G.: Cerebral gigantism. *Pediatrics 41*: 130, 1968.
4. Epstein, C.J., Martin, G.M., Schultz, A.L., and Motulsky, A.G.: Werner's syndrome. *Medicine 45*: 177, 1966.
5. Wertelecki, W., Schindler, A.M., and Gerald P.S.: Partial deletion of chromosone 18. *Lancet 2*: 641, 1966.
6. Elmore, S.M.: Pycnodysostosis, a review. *J. Bone Joint & Surg. 49A:* 153, 1967.
7. Larsen, L.J., Schottstaedt, E.R., and Bost, F.C.: Multiple congenital dislocations associated with characteristic facial abnormalities. *J. Pediat. 37*: 574, 1950.
8. McKusick, V.A., Eldridge, R., Hostelter, J.A., Ruangwit, U., and Eglland, J.A.: Dwarfism in the Amish. II. Cartilage-hair hypoplasia. *Bull. Hopkins Hospital 116*: 285, 1965.
9. Turner, H.H.: A syndrome of infantilism congenital webbed neck and cubitus valgus. *Endrocrinol. 23*: 566, 1938.
10. Smith, D.W.: Autosomal abnormalities. *Am. J. Obstet & Gynec 90*: 1055, 1964.
11. Warkany, J., Passarge, E., and Smith, L.B.: Congenital malformations in autosomal trisomy syndromes. *Am. J. Dis. Children 112*: 502, 1966.
12. Forland, M.: Cleidocranial dysostosis. A review of the syndrome and report of a sporadic case, with hereditary transmission. *Am. J. Med. 33*: 792, 1962.
13. Temtamy, S.A.: Carpenter's syndrome. Acrocephalopolysyndactyly, an autosome recessive syndrome. *J. Pediat. 69*: 111, 1966.
14. Rukavina, J.G., Falls, H.F., Holt, J.F., and Block, W.D.: Leri's pleonosteosis. A study of a family with a review of the literature. *J. Bone Joint & Surg. 41A*: 397, 1959.
15. Blank, C.E.: Apert's syndrome. Observation on British series of 39 cases. *Am. Hum. Genet 24*: 151, 1960.
16. Rubinstein, J.H., and Taybi, H.: Broad thumbs and toes and facial abnormalities. A possible mental retardation syndrome. *Am. J. Dis. Children 105*: 588, 1963.
17. Giroux, J., and Miller, J.R.: Dermatoglyphics of the broad thumb and great toes syndrome. *Am. J. Dis. Children 113*: 207, 1967.
18. Higashi, N., Ikegami, T., and Asada, Y.: Congenital nail defect of index fingers. *Arch. Derm.*: in press, 1977.
19. Konigsmark, B.W.: Hereditary childhood hearing loss and integumentary system disease. *J. Ped. 80*: 909-919, 1972.
20. Mahloudji, M., and Amidi, M.: Simple anonychia. Further evidence for autosomal recessive inheritance. *J. Med. Gene. 8:* 478-480, 1971.
21. Rahbari, H., Heath, L., and Chapel, T.A.: Anonychia with ectrodactyly. *Arch Derm 111*: 1482-1483, 1975.
22. Yesudian,P.,Subranian,P.,andThambiah,A.S.:Anonychiawithectrodactyly.*Arch. Derm.*:inpress, 1977.
23. Basan, M.: Ektodermale dysplasie. Fehlendes papilarmuster, nagelveranderungen und vierfligerfurche. *Arch. Klin. Exp. Derm. 222*: 546, 1965.
24. Clouston, H.R.: The major forms of hereditary ectodermal dysplasia. *Canada Med. Assn. J. 40*: 1, 1939.
25. Warkany, J., Beardry, P.H., and Hornstein, S.: Attempted abortion with 4-amino-pteroglutamic acid (Aminopterin). Malformation of the child. *Am. J. Dis. Child. 97*: 274, 1960.
26. Cole, H.N., Cole, H.N., Jr., and Lascheid, W.D.: Dyskeratosis congenita. Relationship to poikiloderma atrophicans vasculare and to aplastic anemia of Fanconi. *Arch. Derm. 76*: 712, 1957.
27. McKusick, V.A., Egeland, J.A., Eldridge, R., and Krusen, D.E.: Dwarfism in the Amish. The Ellis–Van Creveld syndrome. *Bull. Johns Hopkins Hosp. 115*: 306, 1964.
28. Robinson, G.C., Miller, J.R., and Worth, H.M.: Hereditary enamel hypoplasia. Its association with characteristic hair structure. *Pediatrics 37*: 498, 1966.
29. Feinmesser, M., and Zelig, S.: Congenital deafness with onychodystrophy. *Arch. Otolaryng. 74*: 507, 1961.
30. Holden, J.D., and Akers, W.A.: Goltz syndrome. Focal dermal hypoplasia. A combined mesoectodermal dysplasia. *Am. J. Dis. Child. 114*: 292, 1967.
31. Lowry, R.B., Robinson, G.C., and Miller, J.R.: Hereditary ectodermal dysplasia. Symptoms, inheritance patterns, differential diagnosis and management. *Clin. Pediat. 5*: 395, 1966.
32. Carney, R.G.: Incontinentia pigmenti. A world statistical analysis. *Arch. Derm. 112*: 535-536, 1976.
33. Anderson, I.F.: Maffucci's syndrome. A report of a case with a review of the literature. *S. Afri. Med. J. 39*: 1066, 1965.

34. Lucas, G.L., and Opitz, J.M.: The nail-patella syndrome. Clinical and genetic aspects of 5 kindreds with 39 affected family members. *J. Pediat. 68*: 273, 1966.

35. Gorlin, R.J., Meskin, L.H., and St. Geme, J.W.: Oculodentodigital dysplasia. *J. Pediat. 63*: 69, 1963.

36. Dudding, B.A., Gorlin, R.J., and Langer, L.O.: The oto-palato-digital syndrome. *Am. J. Dis. Child. 113*: 214, 1967.

37. Clarkson, P.: Poland's syndactyly. *Guy's Hosp. Rep. 111*: 335, 1962.

38. Hecht, F., and Jarvinew, J.M.: Heritable dismorphic syndromes with normal intelligence. *J. Pediat. 70*: 927, 1967.

39. Gabr, M., Hashemj, M., Fahmi, A., and Saforth, M.: Progeria. A pathologic study. *J. Pediat. 57*: 70, 1960.

40. Robinson, G.C., Miller, J.R., and Bensimon, J.R.: Familial ectodermal dysplasia with sensorineural deafness and another anomalies. *Pediat. 30*: 797, 1962.

41. Silver, H.K.: Rothmund-Thompson syndrome. An oculocutaneous disorder. *Am. J. Dis. Child. 111*: 182, 1966.

42. Torpin, R.: Fetal malformations caused by amnion rupture. Springfield, Ill.: Charles C. Thomas, 1965.

43. Lagos, J.C., and Gomez, M.G.: Tuberous sclerosis. Re-appraisal of a clinical entity. *Mayo Clinic Proc. 42*: 26, 1967.

44. Warkany, J., Passarge, E., and Smith, L.B.: Congenital malformations in autosomal trisomy syndromes. *Am. J. Dis. Child. 112*: 502, 1966.

45. Reisman, L.E.: Anti-mongolism. Studies in an infant with a partial monosomy of the 21 chromosome. *Lancet 1*: 394, 1966.

46. Qazi, Q.H., and Smithwick, E.M.: Triphalangy of thumbs and great toes. *Am. J. Dis. Child. 120*: 255-257, 1970.

47. Garret, M.J.: Teratogenic effects of combination chemotherapy. *Ann. Int. Med. 80*: 667, 1974.

48. Wilson, R.A., et al: Ankyloglossia superior. *Pediat. 31*: 1051, 1963.

49. Kikychi, I., Hoorikawa, S., and Amano, F.: Congenital (non-hereditary) onychodysplasia of the index fingers (C.O.I.F.). *Arch. Derm. 110*: 743-746, 1974.

50. Higashi, N., Ikegami, T., and Asada, Y.: Congenital nail defect of index fingers (C.O.I.F.). *Arch. Derm.*: in press, 1977.

51. Yesudian, P., Subramanian, P., and Thambiah, A.S.: Anonychia with ectrodactyly. *Arch. Derm.*: in press, 1977.

52. Hundeiker, M.: Hereditare nageldysplasia der 5. zehe. *Der Hautarzt. 20*: 281-282, 1969.

53. Coffin, G.S., and Siris, E.: Mental retardation with absence of fifth fingernail and terminal phalanx. *Am. J. Dis. Child. 119*: 443-439, 1970.

54. Rapp, R.S., and Hodgkin, W.E.: Anhidrotic ectodermal dysplasia. Autosomal dominant inheritance with palate and lip anomalies. *J. Med. Genet. 5*: 269, 1968.

55. Wannarachue, N., Hall, B.D., and Smith, D.W.: Ectodermal dysplasia and multiple defects (Rapp-Hodgkins type). Letter to the Editor. *J. Pediat. 81*: 1217-1218, 1972.

56. Baughman, F.A., Jr.: Chands. The curly hair ankyloblepharon-nail dysplasia syndrome. Skin, hair and nails, birth defects. *Original Articles Series. Vol. VII, No. 8*: 100-102, 1971.

57. Lawrence, R.: Absence of phalanges and toenails. *Med. Radiography and Photography 45*: 46, 1969.

58. Shear, C.S., Nyhan, W.L., Frost, P., and Weinstein, G.D.: Syndrome of unilateral ectromelia, psoriasis and central nervous system anomalies. Skin, hair and nails, birth defects. *Original Article Series, Vol. 8*: 197-203, 1971.

59. Gorlin, R.J., and Sedano, H.: Cryptophthalmia syndrome. *Mod. Med. 1*: 156-157, 1969.

60. Gerald, P.S.: C-type trisomy. *Clin. Lab. Forum.*, Sept. 1969.

61. Sutton-William, G.D.: Keratosis palmo-plantaris variant associated with heliotrichia. *Arch. Klin. Exp. Derm. 236*: 97-106, 1969.

62. Huriez, C., Deminati, M., Agache, P., Delmas-Marsalet, Y., and Menneicer, M.: Sclero-atrophying and keratodermic genodermatosis of the extremities. *Ann. Derm. Syph. (Paris) 96:* 135-146, 1969.

63. Senior, B.: Impaired growth and onychodysplasia. *Am. J. Dis. Child. 122*: 7-9, 1971.

64. Hanson, J.W., and Smith, D.W.: The fetal hydantoin syndrome. *J. Pediat. 87*: 285-290, 1975.

65. Gorlin, R.J., Cohen, M.M., Jr., Wolfson, J.: Tricho-rhino-phalangeal syndrome. *Am. J. Dis. Child. 118*: 595-599, 1969.

66. Warkany, J.: *Congenital Malformations.* Chicago: Year Book Medical Publishers, 1971.

67. McKusick, V.A.: *Heritable Disorders of Connective Tissue.* 3rd ed. St. Louis: C. V. Mosby, 1966.

68. Weary, P.E., Richardson, D.R., Carovati, C.M., and Wood, B.T.: Hereditary sclerosing poikiloderma. *Arch. Derm. 100*: 413-422, 1969.

69. Bergeron, J.R., and Stone, O.J.: Koilonychia. A report of familial spoon nails. *Arch. Derm. 95*: 351-353, 1967.

70. Goodman, R.M., Lockareff, S., and Gwinup, G.: Hereditary congenital deafness with onychodystrophy. *Arch. Otolaryng. 90*: 96-98, 1969.

71. Walbaum, R., Fontaine, G., Lienhardt, J., and Piquet, J.: Surdite familiale avec osteo-onycho-dysplasia. *J. Genet. Hum. 18*: 101-112, 1970.

72. Bart, R.S., and Pumphrey, R.E.: Knuckle pads, leukonychia and deafness. A dominantly inherited syndrome. *N. Eng. J. Med. 276*: 202-205, 1967.

73. Konigsmark, B.W.: Hereditary childhood hearing loss and integumentary system disease. *J. Pediat. 80*: 909-919, 1972.

74. Bushkell, L.L., and Gorlin, R.: Leukonychia totalis, multiple sebaceous cysts and renal calculi. *Arch. Derm. 111*: 899-901, 1975.

75. Baran, R., and Achten, G.: Les associations congenitales de koilonychia et de leuconychie totale. *Arch. Belges Derm. Syph 25*: 13-29, 1969.

76. Albright, S.D., and Wheller, C.E.: Leukonychia. *Arch. Derm. 90*: 392-399, 1964.

77. Lawrence, H.: Leukopathia unguim. *Austr. Med. J. 15*: 483, 1893.

78. Harrington, J.F.: White fingernails. *Arch. Int. Med. 114*: 301-306, 1964.

79. Garrick Wilson, A.: Three cases of hereditary hyperkeratosis of the nail bed. *Brit. J. Derm. 17*: 13-14, 1905.

80. Colcott Fox, T.: Symmetrical hyperkeratosis of the nail beds of the hands and feet and of other areas chiefly on the palms and soles. *Clin. Soc. Trans. (London) 30*: 242-244, 1897.

81. Soderquist, N.A., and Reed, W.A.: Pachyonychia congenita with epidermal cysts and other congenital dyskeratosis. *Arch. Derm. 97*: 31, 1968.

82. Dubowitz, V., Cooke, P., Colver, D., and Harris, F.: Mental retardation, unusual facies and abnormal nails associated with a group-G ring chromosone. *J. Med. Genet. 8*: 195-201, 1971.

83. Wilmont Jacobson, A.: Hereditary dystrophy of the hair and nails. *J.A.M.A.*: 686-689, 1928.

84. Odom, R.B., Stein, K.M., and Maibach, H.I.: Congenital, painful aberrant hyponychium. *Arch. Derm. 110*: 89-90, 1974.

85. Smith, D.W.: Recognizable patterns of human malformations. Philadelphia: W. B. Saunders, 1970.

86. Jadassohn, J., and Lewandosky, F.: Pachyonychia congenita, keratosis disseminata circumscripta; tylomata, leukokeratosis linguae. *Iconograph Derm. Tab. 6*: 29, 1906.

87. Bart, B.J., Gorlin, R.J., Anderson, V.E., and Lynch, F.W.: Congenital localized absence of skin and associated abnormalities resembling epidermolysis bullosa. *Arch. Derm. 93*: 298-304, 1966.

88. Pearson, R.W.: The mechanobullous diseases. In T.B. Fitzpatrick et al. (eds). *Dermatology in General Medicine*. McGraw-Hill, 1971, pp. 621-643.

89. Little, E.M.: Congenital absence or delayed development of the patella. *Lancet 2*: 781-784, 1897.

90. Lucas, G.L., and Opitz, J.M.: The nail patella syndrome. *J. Pediatrics 68*: 273-288, 1966.

91. Simila, S., Vesa, L., and Wasz-Hockert, O.: Hereditary onycho-osteodysplasia (the nail patella syndrome) with nephrosis-like renal disease in a newborn boy. *Pediatrics 46*: 61-65, 1970.

92. Silverman, M.E., Goodman, R.M., and Cupage, F.E.: The nail patella syndrome. *Arch. Int. Med. 120*: 68-74, 1967.

93. Ben-Bassat, M., Cohen, L., and Rosenfeld, J.: The glomellular basement membrane in the nail patella syndrome. *Arch. Path. 92*: 350-355, 1971.

94. Del Pozo, E., and Lapp, H.: Ultrastructure of the kidney in the nephropathy of the nail patella syndrome. *Am. J. Clin. Path. 54*: 845-851, 1970.

95. Linss, G., Hoffmann, G., and Lubs, H.: Nail patella syndrome. Clinical, genetic and biochemical investigations. *Derm. 142*: 145-153, 1971.

96. Thormann, J., and Kobayasi, T.: Pachyonychia congenita, a disorder of keratinization. *Acta Dermatovener (Stockholm) 57*: 63-67, 1977.

97. Danbolt, N., and Closs, K.: Acrodermatitis enteropathica. *Acta Dermatovener 23*: 127-169, 1942.

98. Moynahan, E.J., and Barnes, P.M.: Zinc deficiency and a synthetic diet for lactose intolerance. *Lancet 1*: 676-677, 1973.

99. Wells, B.T., and Winkelmann, R.K.: Acrodermatitis enteropathica. *Arch. Dermat. 84*: 90-102, 1961.

100. Kelley, H et al: Reversible intestinal mucosal abnormality in acrodermatitis enteropathica. *Arch. Dis. Child. 51*: 219-222, 1976.

101. Cash, R., and Berger, C.: Acrodermatitis enteropathica. Defective metabolism of unsaturated fatty acids. *J. Ped. 74*: 717-729, 1969.

102. Ginsburg, R., Robertson, A., and Michel, B.: Acrodermatitis enteropathica. *Arch. Derm. 112*: 653-660, 1976.

103. Nelder, K.H., and Hambridge, K.M.: Zinc therapy in acrodermatitis enteropathica. *New Eng. J. Med. 292*: 879-882, 1975.

104. Dillah, C.J., Lorincz, A.L., and Aavik, O.R.: Acrodermatitis enteropathica. *JAMA 152*: 509-512, 1953.
105. Delves, H.T., Harris, J.T., Lawson, M.S., and Mitchell, J.D.: Zinc and Diodoquin in acrodermatitis enteropathica. *Lancet*: 929, 1975.
106. Endre, L., and Katona, Z.: Etiology of cellular immune deficiency in acrodermatitis enteropathica. *Lancet*: 91, 1976.
107. Amador, M., Pena, M., Garcia-Miranda, A., Gonzales, A., and Hermelo, M.: Low zinc concentrations in acrodermatitis. *Lancet*: 1379, 1975.
108. Walravens, P.A., Hambridge, K.M., Weston, W., and Neldner, K.H.: Plasma zinc in acrodermatitis enteropathica. *Lancet*: 488, 1976.

CHAPTER 6

Surgical Procedures

DIAGNOSTIC AND THERAPEUTIC TECHNIQUES

Through bitter experience, I can state that patients with arterial insufficiency, diabetes or moderate severe DIP (Distal Interphalangeal) arthritis suffer a greater morbidity than any other patients when they undergo surgical manipulation around the nail unit. Infiltration near the MP or CP joints with 1 to 2 cc of anesthetic to each side of the digit is recommended (Fig. 1).

Fingertip Block

A fingertip block can be performed for paring a wart, extracting a foreign body or more complex surgical procedures. The anesthetic should not contain adrenaline or any vasopressor agent; preferably, 2% Lidocaine should be used.

Complete Digital Block

A complete digital block is immediate and lasts 20 minutes. Carbocaine should be used for longer-lasting procedures; it takes 5 to 10 minutes to act and lasts for 1 hour. A 30 gauge needle should be used to infiltrate the skin site where the block is to take place if a larger-bore needle is used later to deliver the anesthetic. Deposition of the local anesthetic along the lateral digital nerve can be done at various points, depending on the desired area of anesthesia.

Partial Block

A partial block can be given laterally on either side of the digit (Fig. 2). The proximal nail fold usually requires its own local infiltration if the block is not at the MP joint level.

In arthritic, diabetic and arterial deficient patients, single injections of local anesthetic around the nail unit often result in moderate pain for days after the procedure. The etiology of this pain is unknown. In digits of children and small toes, a single injection of the anesthetic into the proximal nail fold area further delivers the anesthetic into the dermis of the lunula. The anesthetic will cover all matrix and nail bed areas (Fig. 3). If a tourniquet is used, clamp a large hemostat to it as a reminder to remove it (Fig. 49).

AVULSION OF THE NAIL—SURGICAL

Fig. 2 shows a "grade three" or severly ingrown nail. To avulse the nail, first block the finger as described above, then proceed to separate the nail plate from the proximal nail fold and from its attachment to the underlying nail bed hyponychium. Incisions along the lateral nail fold are not necessary. (See Figs. 4–8 for a pictorial explanation.) Loosen the nail fold (Fig. 4) by inserting a hemostat blade or any other suitable instrument between the horny layer of the proximal nail fold and the nail plate, making sure the toothed portion is against the nail plate. Introduction of the hemostat should always be in a *longitudinal* fashion, *not sweeping transversely across the nail plate*. An instrument that is wider and has no teeth is ideal.[1] A nail plate elevator is available from England,[2] but it is very thick. Once the hemostat is inserted, loosen the attachment of the nail plate and the proximal nail fold by withdrawing and inserting repeatedly in a linear fashion along the entire proximal nail fold (Fig. 5). Similarly, separate the nail plate from the bony layer of the nail bed (Fig. 11; see Chapter 1), inserting the hemostat with the toothed portion against the nail plate, as indicated in Figs. 6 and 7. Do not forget that the distance the hemostat must be inserted is much greater than in the proximal nail groove, since you must go through the entire length of the existing nail plate and then into the most proximal portion of the matrix (Figs. 7, 8).

Again, linear stripping is very important in reducing morbidity and bleeding (Fig. 8). When the nail plate has been completely separated, clamp the hemostat at one lateral edge of the nail plate (Fig. 9) and with a twisting motion rotate the hemostat so as to roll up the now-separated nail plate (Fig. 10). The result is a nice, clean nail bed and a minimal amount of bleeding (Fig. 11).

Usually, the morbidity in this procedure is minimal; bleeding stops by itself. A strip band-aid should be applied along its *longitudinal axis*—NOT around the finger, which could result in a constrictive band with pain later. When the underlying disease is such that there is a great deal of subungal hyperkeratosis, some bleeding may occur during the removal of the nail bed hyperkeratosis since some epithelial avulsions will occur. Again, bleeding is minimal and will stop by itself.

Soaking the area is necessary to maintain a minimum of exudate, usually for 4 to 5 days. A gentle pushing back of the proximal nail fold (arrows up, Fig. 11) is necessary to ensure an "open" (arrows down Fig. 11) proximal nail groove and to prevent "pus" pockets in the proximal nail groove (Fig. 12). Other nail plate avulsion procedures have been described[3] which, in my opinion, carry more morbidity and do not follow anatomically present planes of dissection (Fig. 36).

NAIL BED BIOPSIES

To diagnose tumors or isolated lesions in the nail bed, or when the diagnosis is needed to tell not so much the chronicity of the disease but what the disease is, punch biopsies (Fig. 12) or longitudinal excisions of the nail bed are recommended (Fig. 13). If the overlying nail plate is normal, it must be avulsed prior to obtaining the specimen. If the long-itudinal excision is greater than 2 millimeters, 4-0 or 5-0 dacron or nylon sutures are recommended to close the deficit. Should the nail bed epithelium be very bound down, undermining is required. Morbidity and scarring are usually minimal in minor surgery of the nail bed.

BIOPSIES OF MATRIX AND/OR LUNULA

When pigmented macules or papules or other lesions occur, primarily in the lunula, it is recommended that excision of these lesions be done in a transverse direction (Fig. 14) rather than the longitudinal direction used for the nail bed. Avulsion of the total nail plate again is mandatory (Fig. 15). Some investigators do not avulse the entire nail plate but rather avulse the proximal portion of the nail plate, leaving the distal portion in its place. I believe this will cause a greater morbidity, since edema of the traumatized area will produce a throbbing that does not occur when total avulsion of the nail plate is done. After excision of the lesion of the lunula or matrix (Figs. 16, 17), care must be taken to leave a normal shape to the lunula. It is preferable that sutures not be placed deeply into the dermis (Fig. 18), since in this area the matrix epithelium will become nail plate and will be shed. Thus removal of sutures is not necessary and one can see the sutures emerge from the epithelium of the matrix into the substance of the nail plate as the nail plate is formed and moves distally (Figs. 19, 20). In this fashion, scars of the lunula or matrix are minimized to the greatest potential.

LONGITUDINAL BIOPSY

This procedure is to be done only for investigational purposes, for the correction of a le-sion in the lunula–nail bed area producing a split nail (Fig. 21) or to ascertain the extent of a malignancy. For example, does a squamous cell carcinoma, basal cell carcinoma or Bowen's disease of the nail bed and lunula extend to the joint? In this situation, a long-itudinal biopsy will tell the extent of the invasion of the tumor and its proximity to the joint. This is crucial: if the joint is near invasion, then amputation of the distal digit is nec-essary; by comparison, a local destruction of the surface of the matrix and nail bed does not necessitate amputation. The procedure is as follows:

After suitable digital block, the area of the nail desired for biopsy is isolated prior to ex-cision (longitudinal black and white line, Fig. 21). The sample should be smaller than 3 millimeters in width. For this purpose, the nail plate on both sides of the area to be biop-sied must be avulsed (Figs. 22–28). This is done only when the surgeon desires a biopsy with nail plate; if not, total nail plate avulsion prior to biopsy is recommended. Make sure the nail plate is not separated from the lesion to be biopsied. To avulse those portions of the nail not to be biopsied, insert a small mosquito hemostat carefully (as shown in Fig. 22) to separate the proximal nail fold. Take note that the toothed surface of the hemostat lies against the hard nail plate. Similarly, to separate the nail plate from the nail bed and hyponychium stratum corneum, insert the hemostat with the toothed surface against the nail plate (Fig. 23).

Cut the separated nail on both sides of the island to be biopsied (Figs. 24–28), and with a sharp scalpel excise the 2.5 millimeter (black line) rectangular piece of tissue (Fig. 29). A "crunchy" sensation may be felt while cutting through. This, per se, does not endanger the patient or produce any kind of morbidity; it simply ensures that a good sample is ob-tained. Once the scalpel has outlined the rectangular piece of tissue (Figs. 30, 31), a sharp-curved iris scissor should be introduced to excise the specimen. Make sure that the scissor rests on the bone as the entire length of the piece is excised. In this manner, a rectangular piece of nail biopsy can be obtained (Fig. 32).

The important concept to remember in closing the defect is that the lunula must be approximated and sutured together in such a way as not to leave irregularities in its shape. Make the first suture through the proximal nail fold (arrow, Fig. 33). Then approximate the nail bed (Fig. 34). Sutures should be placed not near the edge of but somewhat away from the incision. This will allow better manipulation of the tissues which may need to be undermined for total approximation. Also, it is important to have the surgical knot away from the incision, as this area may be extremely sensitive at the time of suture removal. Once the lunula has been approximated and the incision closed, no more than 4 or 5 sutures are usually required. The finger is then wrapped with a loose, bulky dressing to ensure a cushion if the patient traumatizes the area. Do not encircle the finger with adhesive, making a constrictive band; rather, spiral the adhesive around the finger. The lesion should be observed for 5 to 7 days, with the sutures removed in approximately 7 days. Little morbidity and deformity are to be expected through this procedure.

AVULSION–NON SURGICAL
OTHER SURGICAL NAIL UNIT PROCEDURES

A review of surgical procedures designed to treat ingrown nail, total destruction of matrix, correction of traumatic nail bed, matrix and digital injuries, and grafting is presented in Figs. 35–46. The author feels that most of the procedures are excessive and result in increased morbidity. It is well to remember that removal of the nail plate decreases morbidity.

MATRIX DESTRUCTION

Phenol[11,12]

After avulsion of the nail plate, it is essential to have a bloodless field. Apply liquid phenol (87 percent) with an applicator into the proximal nail fold to the matrix and paint the area well and with care. After a few minutes, the proximal nail fold should be washed out well and dressed lightly, if at all. Soak the finger and the proximal nail fold. Massage to prevent a matrix abcess, as in the avulsion technique. Morbidity should be 3 to 4 days.

Acrylics and Grafting

Recent work with acrylic nail prosthesis[6] is encouraging. Nail matrix grafting also has been done with good results.[7]

Laser

Recent use of a Sharplan 791 CO_2 laser as a knife has shown promise in the destruction of the matrix area in onychogryphotic nails. Labandter and Kaplan[8] are pioneering this technique and have produced very convincing pictures before and after 6 months of matrix destruction. The technique may become useful in overall nail surgery.

AVULSION—UREA PASTE

This clever procedure takes advantage of the keratolytic action of high concentrations of urea (40%) on the stratum corneum of the nail bed and hyponichium. This, however, limits the therapeutic uses to only those nails which have marked subungual keratosis. It is impossible to avulse nail plates which do not have subungual horn (Fig. 1).

The procedure originated in Russia and was introduced to Western practitioners by Dr. E. Farber. Most of the recorded experience was written by Doctors E. Farber and D. South. (International Psoriasis Bulletin 5:3, 1978.)

Procedure: The surface of the skin around the nail can be painted with tincture of Benzoin. Cover all the skin surface surrounding the nail plate which is to be avulsed with a suitable adhesive material, such as plastic film wrap. Apply the 40% urea paste to the surface of and under the nail plate. Then cover the nail plate with a material such as was used to cover the surrounding skin. (I prefer to soak the finger or toe nail for twenty minutes prior to this procedure.) In three to seven days, the nail and subungual debris will look white and will be easily debrided. The procedure is basically trouble free. Remember this does not work for normal nails.

GENERAL OBSERVATIONS FOLLOWING SURGERY OR OTHER PROCEDURES

Edema

As a result of the surgical procedure, the fingertip swells. This may result in vague sensations that make the patient aware of the finger. Aspirin or phenacetin usually gives adequate control. Hand elevation and use of a cloth sling for 2 to 4 hours immediately after surgery minimizes morbidity.

Soaks

Whenever the nail unit is devoid of epithelium, either in avulsions or excisions, and bleeding or oozing occurs, soaking is necessary in order to reduce the bacterial flora on the surgical or denuded area. Soaking in saline or any preferred water solution twice a day until oozing ceases (usually for 5 days) will ensure a clean surface.

Dressings

Minor nail unit surgical procedures, such as avulsion or small biopsies, should not have a large bulky dressing but rather a strip band-aid applied longitudinally to the wound (Fig. 35). It is important to apply the band-aid loosely so that air and water can pass between the band-aid and the surface of the digit. If the band-aid is too tight, throbbing usually occurs at the tip of the finger. Band-aids can be changed daily.

After large surgical procedures, such as longitudinal biopsies or deep excisions with suturing, a bulky dressing should be applied to the fingertip. This dressing should have Telfa in opposition to the skin, followed by shock-proof dressing such as Curlex or other bandaging material, and should all be held together by either a stocking or adhesive tape. The stocking or tape is applied in a spiraling fashion from the fingertip to the base of the finger, so as not to encircle the finger at any one point. This will allow for swelling and will eliminate the throbbing commonly seen when dressings are too tight.

Throbbing

As stated previously, throbbing results from edema and dressings that are too tight. Elevation of the finger shortly after surgery for 2 to 4 hours or so assumes adequate edema drainage; if the dressing is not too tight, this drainage will occur freely, producing no throbbing.

Sharp Pain

This usually denotes a very tight suture holding the skin or a suture which is in or very near the periosteum. This suture may be removed if the pain does not stop within 24 to 48 hours.

Supportive Care

The patient should be given a prescription of 30 milligrams of codeine, if not allergic, or another moderate analgesic to be carried with him in the event that trauma occurs to the operated finger.

Adhesion

Nonadherent gauze may be inserted into the proximal nail fold space after avulsion to prevent adhesion.

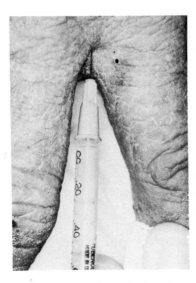

Fig. 1. Injection of anesthetic at base of finger. Introduce needle at least 1/4 inch into skin.

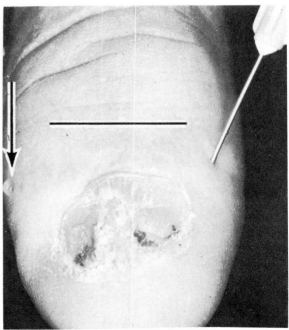

Fig. 2. Fingertip or nail unit block with anesthetic directed to lateral nerves. In this procedure the proximal nail fold is not anesthetized and must be locally infiltrated (transverse line).

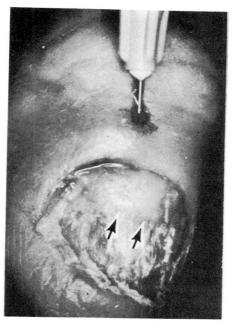

Fig. 3. Technique for blocking fingers of small children or toes. Obliquely through the proximal nail fold, pass matrix into dermis of lunula/nail bed.

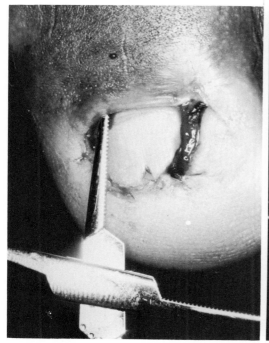

Fig. 4. Large toenail with grade III ingrown nail. Note that granulation tissue covering medial aspect of nail plate has developed own epithelial cover.

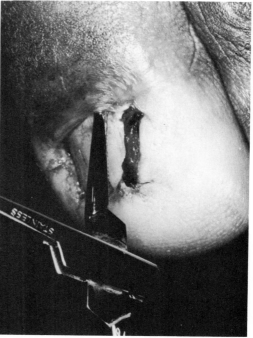

Fig. 5. To avulse nail, first insert toothed portion of hemostat in proximal nail fold against nail plate. Movement should be longitudinal and distal, not across surface of nail plate.

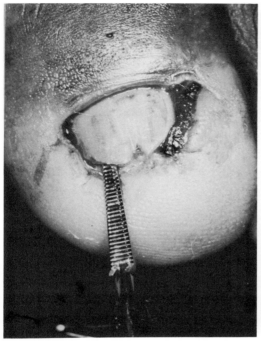

Fig. 6. Another stripping of proximal nail fold, again by longitudinal and distal insertion.

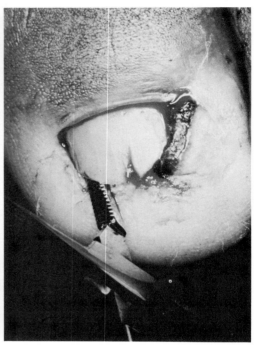

Fig. 7. Insertion of toothed portion of hemostat undrneath nail plate, so that stripping of nail plate will be proximal distally.

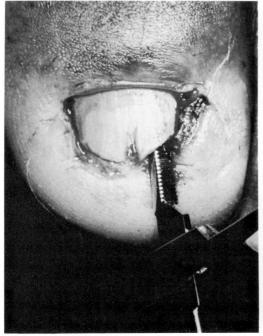

Fig. 8. Hemostat inserting greater distance than in proximal nail fold stripping.

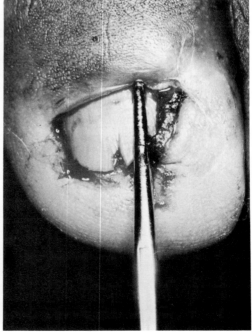

Fig. 9. Complete separation of nail plate from nail bed by stripping entire surface in longitudinal distal fashion.

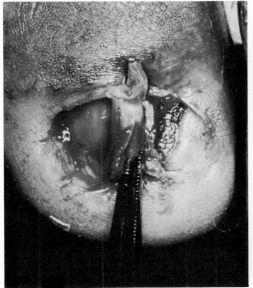

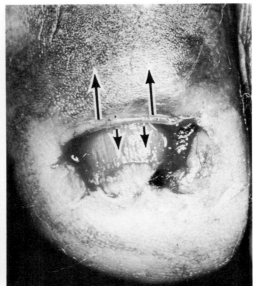

Fig. 10. After nail plate has been separated, clamp hemostat at one end of nail plate near lateral border, as in Fig. 8; with twisting motion, peel off nail plate.

Fig. 11. End results of avulsion of nail plate.

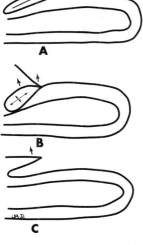

Fig. 12. Diagrammatic drawing of how to prevent proximal nail fold pseudo-abscess after nail plate avulsion. (A) Represents space created by avulsion (long arrow). (B) Edema tends to close space creating a pseudo-abscess (crossed arrows). (C) This can be prevented with marriage of PNF proximally (arrow up) thus keeping opened the proximal nail groove.

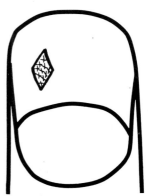

Fig. 14. Diagrammatic drawing of direction of excision in nail bed area. Compare to transverse direction in matrix (Fig. 17).

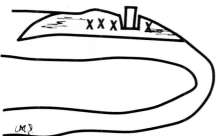

Fig. 13. Diagrammatic drawing of use of punch biopsy in diagnosis of tumor.

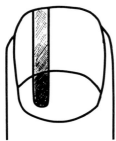

Fig. 15. Diagrammatic drawing of pigmented lesion in lunula. Also, pigmenting nail plate.

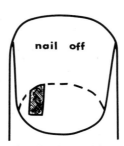

Fig. 16 After avulsion of nail plate.

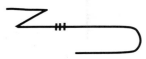

Fig. 19. Profile of finger in Fig. 18 following matrix repair.

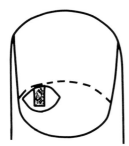

Fig. 17. Transverse excision of pigmented lesion. This procedure will leave no scar.

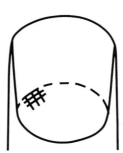

Fig. 18. Sutured matrix.

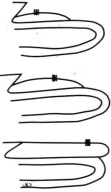

Fig. 20. Sequence of sutures as new nail plate grows out. Sutures need not be taken out if placed superficially.

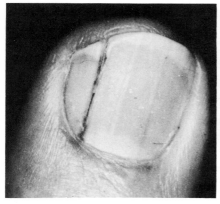

Fig. 21. Split nail plate in thumb. No history of trauma. Nail should be avulsed first; if defect returns longitudinal excisions will correct it.

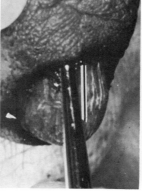

Fig. 22. Sequence to obtain longitudinal nail unit sample for biopsy or to correct defect in Fig. 21. Separation of proximal nail fold from nail plate.

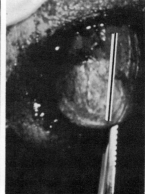

Fig. 23. Separation of nail plate from nail bed hyponychium.

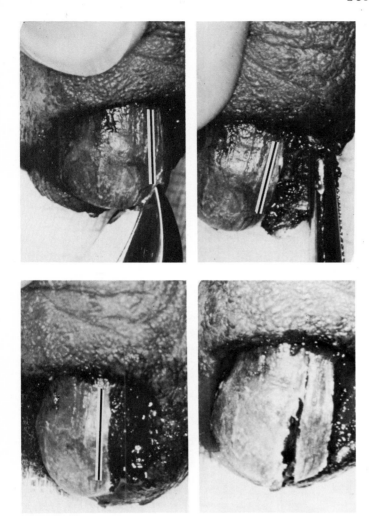

Fig. 24, 25, 26, 27. Avulsion of nail plate on both sides of area to be biopsied if sample desired is to have nail plate. If sample with nail plate not desired, avulse total nail plate.

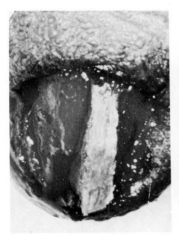

Fig. 28 Isolation of area to be biopsied.

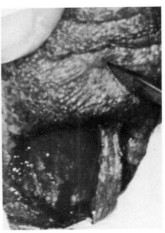

Fig. 29 Scalpel outline of rectangular area to be biopsied.

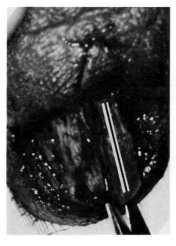
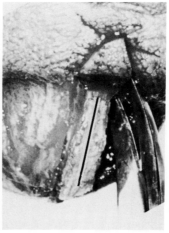
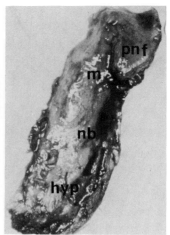

Fig. 30 Fig. 31 Excision of specimen with iris scissors.

Fig. 32 Nail biopsy. (Note matrix, M; nail bed, NB; and hyponychium, HYP.

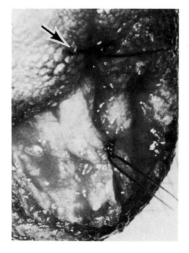
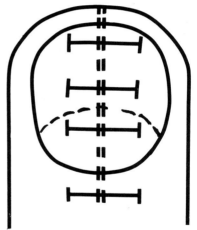

Fig. 33. Note suture (arrow) through proximal nail fold, *not* matrix.

Fig. 34. Final suture pattern leaves all structures in normal relationship. Undermining may be necessary. Note wide placement of sutures to incision line.

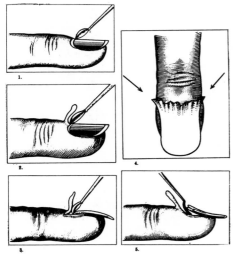

Fig. 35. Cordero's[3] nail plate avulsion. Excessive morbidity.

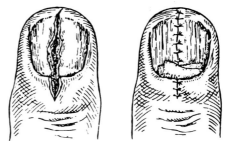

Fig. 36. Single repair of lacerations. Nail plate off.

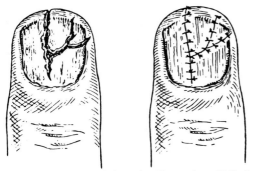

Fig. 37. Compounded repair of lacerations. Nail plate off.

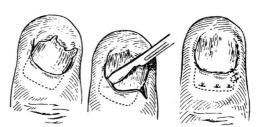

Fg. 38. Repair of irregular matrix.

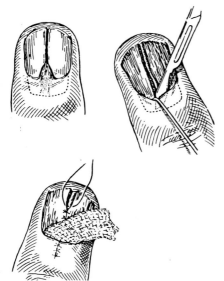

Fig. 39 Correction of pterygium.

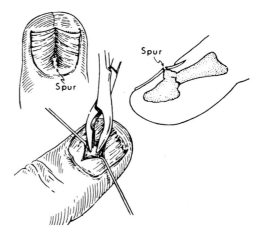

Fig. 40 Removal of exostosis. Digital block at metacarpal phalangeal and carpal phalangeal joint area.

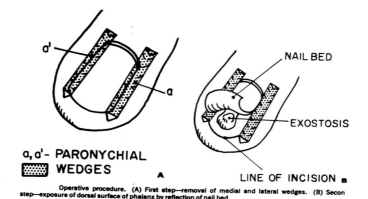

a, a'- PARONYCHIAL WEDGES

NAIL BED

EXOSTOSIS

LINE OF INCISION

Operative procedure. (A) First step—removal of medial and lateral wedges. (B) Secon step—exposure of dorsal surface of phalanx by reflection of nail bed.

Fig. 41. Removal of exostosis.

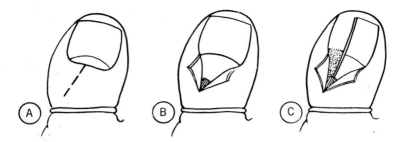

Winograd's operation. [A] *Line of incision;* [B] *exposure of nail root;* [C] *involved part of nail removed. Shaded area shows extent of matrix ablation after partial nail removal.*

Fig. 42. Winograd's partial matrix removal.

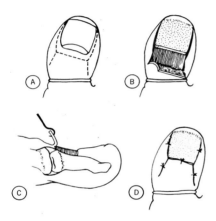

Zadik's operation. [A] *Line of incision;* [B] *flap lifted and phalanx exposed after matrix ablation;* [C]. *extent of matrix ablation;* [D] *flaps sutured to edge of sterile nail bed.*

Fig. 43. Total matrix removal. Zadik's procedure.

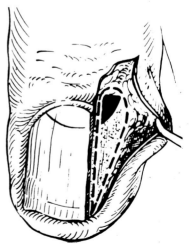

Fig. 44. Partial matrix procedure. Excellent matrix visualization.

Fig. 45.

Recurrence Rates

	I Ablation of Nail Bed	II Ablation of Nail Bed with Shortening of Phalanx	III Watson- Cheyne Operation	Zadik's Operation
Recurrence rate	31%	30%	85%	73%
Total ablations	26	10	7	26

Fig. 45 Chart comparing regrowth of nail spicules after various matrix removal procedures.

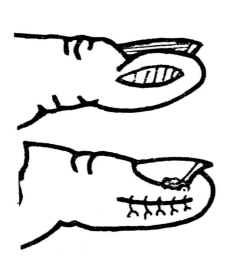

Fig. 46 Excisions of "granulomatous paronychia" to correct ingrown nail.

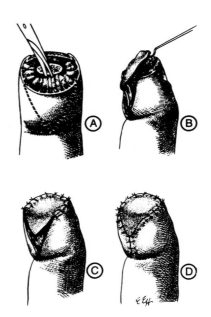

Kleinert method for repair of fingertip amputations. (A) Triangular flap of skin is incised and mobilized. (B) Triangular flap is advanced over the smoothed bone end. (C) Base of flap is sutured to the nail bed, and (D) defect is closed by the V-Y technique.

Fig. 47 Plastic correction of fingertip injuries. Kleinert's method.

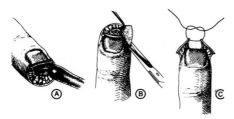

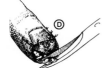

Kutler method for repair of fingertip amputations. (A) Sharp corners are rounded to provide normal contour and to prevent impingement on the pulp. (B) Triangular flaps are developed and mobilized with small plastic scissors while traction is applied with a skin hook. (C) The flaps are sutured together, (D) excess pulp is removed, and (E) the closure is completed.

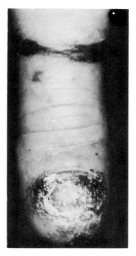

Fig. 48 Plastic correction of fingertip injuries. Kutler's method.

Fig. 49. Tourniquet left on for 24 hours after surgery. Fortunately only minor damage to skin resulted.

NOTES

1. Albon, M.J.: Surgical gems avulsion of a nail plate. *J. Derm. Surg. Oncol. 3*: 34-35, 1977.

2. McKay, I.: Nail elevator. *Lancet H*: 864, 1973.

3. Cordero, F.A.: Ablación ungueal. *Derm. Int.14*: 21-26, 1965.

4. Fulp, M.: New enzyme aids phenol technique in nail surgery. *Podiatry Assoc. 62*: 395-398, 1972.

5. Wee, G.C., and Tucker, G.L.: Phenolic cauterizations of the matrix in the surgical cure of ingrown nails. *Miss. Med. 66*: 802-803, 1969.

6. Bautista, B.N., and Nery, E.B.: Replacement of a malformed fingernail with acrylic resin material. *Plas. & Reconstructive Surg. 55*: 234-236, 1975.

7. McCash, C.R.: Free nail grafting. *Brit. J. Plas. Surg. 8*: 19-33, 1955.

8. Labandter, H., and Kaplan, I.: Experience with a "continuous" laser in the treatment of suitable cutaneous conditions: preliminary report. *J. Dermatol. Surg. Oncol. 3*: 527-530, 1977.

9. Kleinert, H.E., Putcha, S.A., Ashbell, T.S., and Kutz, J.E.: The deformed fingernail. A frequent result of failure to repair nail bed injuries. *J. Trauma 7*: 177-189, 1967.

10. Winograd, A.M.: A modification in the technique of operations for ingrown toenails. *JAMA 92*: 229, 1929.

11. Zadik, F.R.: Obliterations of the nail bed without shortening of terminal phalanx. *J. Bone & Joint Surg. 32B*: 66, 1950.

12. Krull, E.A.: Cited in *Derm. in Practice 6*: 1974.

13. Lloyd-Davies, R.W.: Nail bed ablation. *Brit. J. Surg. 50*: 44-46, 1962.

14. Jemec, B., and Anderson, J.E.: Surgical treatment of paronychia granulomatosa hallices. *Acta Dermato. Vener. (Stockholm) 55*: 319-320, 1975.

15. Kutler, W.: A new method for fingertip amputations. *JAMA 133*: 29-30, 1947.

CHAPTER 7

Ingrown Nails

Ingrown nails regularly occur in toenails and are rarely seen in the fingers. Anatomically and pathologically, the process should be considered similar to that of ingrown hairs.

An ingrown nail occurs when the nail plate pierces or is about to pierce the lateral fold epithelium and there is "commerce" between the keratinous nail plate and the LNF dermal elements (Figs. 1, 2). Clinically, this involves three stages; these are identified since treatment is different for each stage (Figs. 3–5).

CAUSES

1. Uneven cutting or tearing (Fig. 1) of the nail plate, a favorite pastime, will result in a temporary abutment of the lateral nail fold (LNF) to the edge of the plate and set the stage for penetration of the plate through the LNF epithelium.

2. Disease states which result in abnormal nail plate changes, as in onychomycosis and dystrophies, may foster the piercing of the LNF by the nail plate.

Clinical Stages

Stage I: The earliest signs and symptoms of ingrown nails are pain, slight swelling, and hyperhydrosis of the area involved. The nail plate has injured the LNF epidermis (Figs. 2, 3, 5, 6), resulting in a series of events that produce edema. The edema aggravates the condition by causing further compression of the underlying dermal tissue between the hard nail plate and the bony phalanx. Varying degrees of sweelling and redness may occur, depending on the age of the dermal insult. Treatment consists of the stepwise extraction of the intruding nail plate from the dermis of the LNF by elevation of the nail plate with the introduction of as much nonabsorbent cotton as possible under the area of the nail plate involved (arrow, Figs. 4, 5; Chap. 10, Fig. 7). Generally, there is some pain, but the patient himself, once instructed, will pack more cotton than the physician can. This should be removed daily and repacked, always with the maximum amount possible. Usually, 7 to 14 days is necessary to correct the situation.

Stage II: This is characterized by exquisitely sharp pain, hyperhydrosis and the formation of granulation tissue arising from the LNF dermis through the new "broken" or ulcerated LNF epidermis growing over the nail plate, fixing it in place (Figs. 8–11). The LNF is very edematous, and constant seropurulent exudation is present. A fetid odor, produced by colonization of colonic or gram-positive bacteria on the surface of the granulating tissue, may accompany this stage. By and large, no systemic antibiotics are needed; however, soaks can be beneficial in reducing the number of surface bacteria. Pressure from shoes or other footwear is pain-producing.

Surgical intervention should not be the first choice of treatment. The granulation tissue can be dramatically reduced in 1 or 2 days by application of high-potency steroids, steroid tape or intralesional corticosteroid injections (10 mg/cc triacinolone acetonide). Once the granulation tissue is gone, the nail plate is no longer fixed and treatment with cotton, as in stage I, can be started.

Stage III: Symptomatically, this stage is similar to stage II, but anatomically there is one very important difference. The granulation tissue over the nail plate is covered on its surface by epidermis, making it impossible for the nail plate to be elevated out of the LNF groove (Figs. 12, 13) without the aid of surgical intervention. Avulsion of the entire nail plate (as shown in Chapter 5) is recommended. The granulating mass may be cauterized or excised.

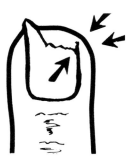

Fig. 1. Diagrammatic drawing of events leading to ingrown nails. External forces due to **shoe-clad environment** (thick double arrows) push LNF into distally moving and irregularly shaped (pointed) nail plate (thick arrow up).

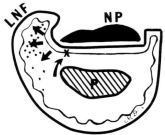

Fig. 2. Diagrammatic drawing of cross-section of events in Fig. 1. Nail plate (NP) pushes into lateral nail fold (LNF) (3 arrows same direction) and produces edema (dots). X marks area under NP where, if sufficient cotton is packed, nail plate will elevate over LNF.

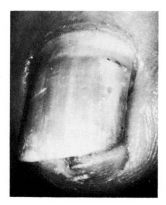

Fig. 3. Clinical stage I, ingrown nail.

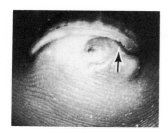

Fig. 4. Stage II, ingrown nail (arrows point to where cotton should be packed).

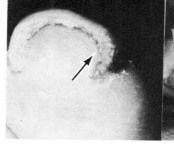

Fig. 5. Laterally compressed toenails, common cause of ingrown nails. Stage I.

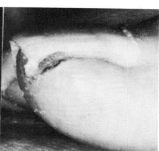

Fig. 6. Side view of Fig. 5.

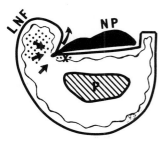

Fig. 7. Once nail plate pierces LNF, dermal elements react to NP as foreign body with resulting edema and cellular infiltrate. This starts series of events resulting in exquisite pain and granulation of tissue eventually extending beyond LNF (arrow up). X marks site where cotton can still elevate NP over LNF.

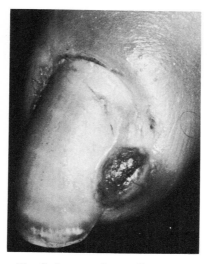

Fig. 8. Ingrown fingernail, uncommon site, usually follows tearing of LNF cuticle.

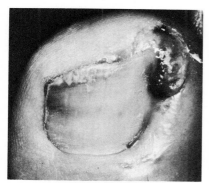

Fig. 9. Stage II, ingrown toenail, granulation tissue over nail plate.

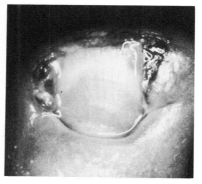

Fig. 10. Bilateral ingrown toenail. Stage II.

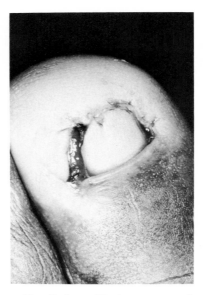

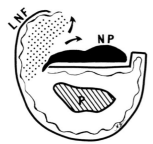

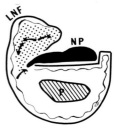

Fig. 11. Stage II, ingrown nail. Granulation tissue may become exuberant and fix nail plate in "ingrown" position. Treatment depends on eliminating granulation tissue and reverting to stage I.

Fig. 12 Stage III, ingrown toenail. Epidermis covers granulation tissue, usually sign of long-term disease.

Fig. 13. Stage III. With time, epidermis of LNF overgrows longstanding "proud flesh," making treatment of this condition difficult by means other than surgery.

CHAPTER 8

Onychomycosis

Onychomycosis is defined as the infection of the nail unit by fungi. The terms *tinea ungium* and *nail ringworm* were used as synonyms when onychomycosis was thought to be produced exclusively by dermatophytic fungi. Today, however, nondermatophytic fungi and yeast, as well as dermatophytes, are known to be agents of onychomysis. The terms mentioned above should be discouraged since they bring confusion to the medical literature. The more precise terms *dermatophytic, nondermatophytic* and *yeast onychomycosis* are recommended.

CLINICAL TYPES

Four clinical types of onychomycosis are recognized by the manner in which the nail plate is invaded by fungi. Each represents a different host-parasite relationship (Fig. 1).[1] The four types are: distal subungual (Fig. 2), white superficial (Fig. 3), proximal subungual (Fig. 4) and Candida albicans (Fig. 5).

Distal Subungual Onychomycosis (DSO) (Fig. 2)

In this clinical type, the most commonly seen, the causal organism first invades the nail unit by gaining access to the hyponychial horny layers (single arrow, Fig. 2). As the infection continues, the underside of the nail plate is involved (double arrow, Fig. 2); in the later stages of the disease, the nail plate undergoes color and texture changes (Figs. 6, 7, 10), resulting in complete changes in the appearance of the nail. Various causal agents change the nail plate in a characteristic fashion, and there is a variable time in the extent of nail invasion. As the infection progresses, the subungual debris, consisting of hyponychial and nail bed stratum corneum, provides a nidus where other organisms can settle and thrive. This, in turn, adds to the changing of the chemical-physical properties of the nail plate's underside (see Diagnostic Considerations). Eventually, the nail plate separates from the nail bed (Fig. 8, 9) and either crumbles off or is cut off by the patient. The entire nail plate may be off the fingertip, showing only the hyperkeratotic nail bed (Fig. 10).

Histopathologically, the fungal hyphae (arrow, Fig. 4) are seen in the stratum corneum of the nail bed and in the hyponychium. The fungal elements are characteristically long hyphae. The epidermis may show typically focal spongiosis with overlying focal parakeratosis. There is a superficial inflammatory response of the upper dermis.

Finger DSO is exclusively the result of dermatophytic infections. Virtually all these fungi have been reported to produce this disease (see Table I). On a world-wide basis, T. rubrum and T. mentagrophytes are the most commonly reported. Characteristically, these organisms invade the nail plate and produce a whitish streaking pattern described by earlier investigators under such names as the "transverse" and the "springy" networks[2,3] (arrow, Fig. 7).

Nondermatophytic Fungi

In the toenails, the causative agents are more varied, with nondermatophytic fungi rarely occurring (see Table II). Although fungi have been reported to be pathogens, certain cephalosporiums, *fusarium oxysporum* and certain aspergilli occur more frequently than any other nondermatophytic organisms (Figs. 12, 13). Criteria for pathogenicity in the nondermatophytes are (1) the presence of hyphal forms in the infected subungual debris, (2) the persistent failure to culture recognized dermatophytes and (3) the regularity of cultures of these nondermatophytes (see Table III). The treatment of DSO relies on knowing the causal agent (see Diagnostic Considerations and Therapy). Yeasts have also been incriminated as agents of DSO,[4] and, most commonly, C. albicans and C. parapsilosis are recovered from onycholytic nails and mixed dermatophyte yeast infections (Table IV; Fig. 11). C. albicans is accepted as a pathogen, but C. parapsilosis is not. Table IV correlates hyphae in nails with cultures showing C. parapsilosis producing pseudohyphae in the abnormal toenail. C. parapsilosis is so commonly recovered from "wet" skin surfaces that some investigators consider it normal flora.

Distal Subungual Onychomycosis with Other Dermatologic Diseases

Patients with Hansen's disease often have DSO. Patients with systemic fungal disease may have an onychomycotic clinical picture resulting from the nail unit invasion by the deep mycotic agent; examples are chromomycosis and coccidioidomycosis. Patients on long-term systemic corticosteroids often have widespread body and nail dermatophytosis.

Dermatophytic fungal infection of nails affected with Darier's (Figs. 16, 17), lichen planus (Figs. 18–20) and ichthyotic states can coexist. In psoriatic toenails (Figs. 14, 15), psoriasis and fungal infection may occur.[49] Psoriatic fingernails usually are involved with C. albicans rather than with dermatophytosis.

White Superficial Onychomycosis (WSO) (Fig. 3)

This clinical entity occurs exclusively in toenails. It is very common and usually goes unnoticed because it produces little symptomatology and barely destroys the nail plate.

The causal agent invades the superficial surface of the nail plate. Penetration of the nail plate is minimal. Clinically, these small foci of invasion look like white islands (Fig. 3), which may measure smaller than 1 millimeter and may coalesce to form larger patches (Figs. 26, 27). The clinical picture was first described by Jessner,[5] who, assuming it was caused only by fungus of the genus Trichophyton, named it leukonychia trichophytica. The most common organisms, however, are *T. mentogrophytes* and, of late, *Microsporum persicolor.* WSO is also produced by *Fusarium oxysporum* and Cephalosporium (Figs. 21–26) and Aspergilli (Figs. 27–30). The colonies of *T. mentagrophytes* and *Microsporum persicolor* are often clinically confused. Table V describes the causal agents in this condition. It is interesting to note that *T. rubrum* has not been noted to produce this clinical onychomycotic entity, even though it is one of the most common causative agents for onychomycosis. Only recently has *T. rubrum* been reported to be a causative agent of WSO,[6] and this needs further confirmation.

Histopathologically, this condition is rather unique in that the organism is seen in the nail plate not as long hyphal forms (as in skin dermatophytosis and DSO) but rather in forms of the fungal saprophytic state (Figs. 22–25). Short, gnarled fungal bodies, which English[7] refers to as eroding fronds or carpal bodies, are the usual morphology (Figs. 24, 25, 30). This is the case regardless of the organism producing the clinical disease.

Proximal Subungual Onychomycosis (PSO) (Fig. 4)

Typical of the fingernails and by far the rarest of all onychomycoses, this type starts as a leukonychic spot (arrows, Figs. 31, 32) on the proximal portion of the nail plate. At first, it looks like an ordinary white spot resulting from manipulation of the cuticle area, but it may progress into a plaque which is distinctly under the surface of the nail plate (arrow, Figs. 33, 34). Eventually, the entire nail may be affected.

There may be intervals of normal nail plate (Figs. 31 and 32). One must have a high index of suspicion or the diagnosis of onychomycosis will not be made. A small sample of the nail plate should be prepared for direct microscopy and culture. The paucity of reports precludes general statements on the causal agents, but personally I have seen four cases, all by *T. rubrum.* Also implicated are T. megninii and Èpidermorphytom floccosum.[8] The treatment is by Griseofulvin, as in DSO. The causal agent penetrates through the proximal nail fold (Figs. 33, 35). In the proximal nail fold, a normal dermatophytic histopathologic picture is produced (Fig. 35). The fungus limits its growth to the ventral aspect of the nail (arrow, Figs. 33, 34).

Candida Onychomycosis (Fig. 5)

This type of onychomycosis is seen only in patients who suffer from chronic muco-cutaneous candidiasis and other immunologic cellular states. It affects fingernails and toenails (Figs. 36, 44, 45). Usually, invasion of the nail plate is from the hyponychial horn, but the yeast rapidly invades the entire thickness of the nail plate and moves proximally to involve the length of the plate (Figs. 37, 38). At a quick glance, it looks like DSO except that it involves the entire thickness of the plate. The thickened nail plate sits on an abnormal digit tip, which is rather bulbous but not clubbed (Figs. 44, 45). The nail plate eventually becomes very dystrophic and appears to be greatly destroyed (Fig. 46). The nail involvement clinically resembles that seen in keratotic (Norwegian) scabies. Direct microscopic examination will reveal many hyphal forms (Fig. 39, 40)—eroding fronds as well as the typical yeast forms seen in candida infections (Figs. 41–43). Hanser and Rothman[9] studied many strains of *C. albicans* from patients who had the usual syndrome and found no basic difference among the yeast strains; perhaps the nail plates of these patients are chemically different.

Histologically, interesting changes are seen in the fungal forms which the yeast exhibits in the nail plate. The hyphae are similar to those seen in Candida albicans invasion of the central nervous system (brain) (Figs. 39, 43). The entire thickness of the nail plate is invaded by the pseudo-hyphae. The epidermis of the matrix nail bed and hyponychium show spongiosis, and there is a mild perivascular inflammatory reaction in the dermis (Fig. 40). No yeast cells or granulonatous reaction is noted in the dermis; the term *candida granuloma* should be disregarded.

DIAGNOSTIC CONSIDERATIONS

Fungal disease presents a unique situation in·that once a characteristic fungal element is demonstrated by direct microscopy, the diagnosis is confirmed. In onychomycosis, however, the nail plate provides difficulties in handling, clearing and culturing. The preferred site for the demonstration of fungal elements is where they abound:

1. In DSO, one must pick the softer subungual debris, not the nail plate; preferably, material should be obtained that does not come off easily but must be picked from under the nail plate (arrows, Fig. 2).

2. In WSO., material should come superficially from the whitish areas of the nail plate (arrow, Fig. 3).

3. In PSO, one must pare down the normal surface of the nail plate and then obtain material which is white from the deeper portions of the plate (arrows down, Fig. 31).

4. In candida onychomycosis, material may come from any place where the nail plate looks abnormal (arrow, Figs. 37, 38).

Clearing the Specimen for Direct Microscopy

The improved formulaion of potassium hydroxide and dimethysulfoxide is a definite advantage in nail specimens.[10]

1. Prepare a 20% KOH solution (20 g KOH in 100 cc H_2O).

2. Mix 60 cc of the 20% KOH solution with 40 cc pure DMSO, technical grade.

The presence of a long hyphal element probably means that the particular fungus is growing in the nail material. Hyphae are usually colorless (dermatophytes and most nondermatophytes) but could be tan-brown. The tan-brown hyphae are nondermatophytic agents, recently described, which are capable of producing a clinical picture of tinea pedis and onychomycosis (DSO) (Fig. 13). They are fungi of the genera Hendersonula[11] and Scytalidium.[12] Neither grows in actidione-containing media such as mycosel or DTM (dermatophyte test medium).

Selection of a Culture Medium

A culture medium is devised to allow the growth of predetermined organisms or a selective flora. Generally, in dermatology, two types of media are used: (1) the universal media (Sabouraud's), which allows all organisms of interest to the dermatologist, e.g., yeasts, molds, dermatophytes and some bacteria, to grow (Figs. 47, 48) (the hazard of using such a medium is shown by the up-arrows in Figs. 47 and 48, where the bacteria present overgrow the medium faster than the other organisms present, or it may be that the bacteria produce an inhibitory substance against the fungus meant to be isolated) and (2) selective media containing a series of antibiotics to suppress bacteria and molds but which allow the growth of yeast and nondermatophytes (commonly used are Mycosel without a color indicator and dermatophyte test medium with a color indicator;[13] these cycloheximide-containing media will not allow the recovery of fungi such as Hendersonula and Scytalidium capable of onychomycosis, tinea pedis and tinea palmaris). For further explanation, see descriptions of Figs. 47 and 48.

Discrepancy Between Direct Demonstration of Fungal Element and Recovery from Culture

Many explanations have been written by many authors about the discrepancy between direct positive and culture negative nails: failure to use fancy homogenizers, nail drills, grinders, etc., to release the fungus or failure to use special culture medias and the like.

Personally, I don't know why this occurs; my own recovery rate is about 80 percent. Another possible explanation for seeing the fungus but not growing it is that the causal agent is dead. I have studied a few cases of DSO in which a micrococcus was present and produced an antifungal agent which inhibited the growth of the fungus *in vivo*. This micrococcus must live for a short period of time in the subungual debris; otherwise, the nail would self-heal. The coesisting micrococcus can inhibit microsporum and trichophyton species (Fig. 49).

Discussion of Subungual Onychomycosis

This clinical entity presents interesting facets which I would like to briefly touch upon. For a moment, let us consider onychomycosis by *T. rubrum*. Is this not one of the most common causal agents? If so, why does it not produce WSO? Could it be that *T. rubrum* is not as capable a nail invader as we think? Is it making a living in DSO as the result of efforts from a coexisting organism? Why is T. mentagraphytes unique in being the causal agent in WSO? Is T. mentagrophytes better suited biochemically to invade the nail plate than *T. rubrum*? *Pseudomonas aeurginosa*, on the other hand, is well accepted by clinicians as a nail destroyer. Clinically, onychomycosis with Pseudomonas creates a large subungual space. The space created by the subungual debris, beneath the nail plate, is a nidus where, microbiologically, a varied number of organisms are found. Do any of these organisms contribute to the destruction of the nail plate? And, if so, which ones? To answer these questions, the following experiments were done.

The organisms found in 10 toenails with DSO were cultured and identified. They consisted of gram-positive micrococci, Pseudomonas, Candida albicans, C. parapsilosis, dermatophytes, and a host of nondermatophytic fungi. No attempt was made to culture for streptomyces, actinomyces or mycobacteria. The experiment consisted of growing various onychomycotic-isolated organisms in a medium containing radioactive nail plate and measuring the amount of nail breakdown by the amount of radiolabel releasing from the nail plate by the organism breakdown capabilities. The plan was to prepare a substrate which would mimic the *in vivo* human nail situation. Monkey nail plate was used.

Injections of ^{14}C-cystine were made intralesionally near the matrix in the monkeys' fingers. After a suitable time period, these nail plates were avulsed, finely cut, washed out and pooled into 3 mg aliquots. These clippings were bagged in nylon sacks to prevent their dispersion and washed until all the soluble radioactivity was eliminated (Fig. 50) and only that incorporated as nail protein was left. A number of these 3 mg aliquots of nail plate were "burned," and the $14-CO_2$ was collected and measured. Because the nail clippings were pooled and the amounts of radioactivity were fairly constant, a total amount of radioactivity could be determined for each 3 mg nail aliquot.

Various organisms were then cultured in a rich medium with the radiolabeled nail for 3 weeks. At the end of the period, the sack of nails, the organisms and the medium were prepared accordingly and the radioactivity released by each organism was tabulated: Fig. 51 shows these results. It is clear, as in the clinical situation, that *Pseudomonas aeruginosa* is the best nail destroyer. *T. mentagrophytes* is next best and far below are *T. rubrum* and other nail-associated fungi, yeast and bacteria, including the microccocus which produces an antifungal chemical.

It has always been said, rather than proven, among dermatologists that *T. rubrum* infections are slow and very chronic. It may on the basis of hard fact that this clinical experience occurs.

THERAPY

One must consider the causal agent in the treatment of onychomycosis, since dermatophytic fungi are sensitive to Griseofulvin and the nondermatophytes are not. In addition, dermatophytic onychomycosis usually reinfects from a plantar-palmar reservoir, while nondermatophytic fungi do not usually have such a reservoir simple ovulsion sufficing for a cure. An exception is Hendersonula tortuloidea, a nondermatophyte which produces Tinea pedis and T. palmaris as well as onychomycosis.

Of great promise is the recent introduction in the antifungal field of chemicals which are considered broad-spectrum in activity. These compounds have been tested as topical medications and are effective against Candida and dermatophytes but not against nondermatophytes. Since the bulk of the onychomycotic disease is produced by dermatophytic fungi, adequate therapy exists today.

In spite of the recent advances, the fact remains that the treatment of choice for dermatophytic onychomycosis is systemic Griseofulvin. First, special situations will be discussed. The greatest promise in the systemic antimycotic therapy is ketoconazole.

Treatment of White Superficial Onychomycosis

As stated previously, this infection is superficial on the nail plate; therefore, many chemicals can penetrate the superficial layers of the nail plate and cure the infection. Mechanical scraping of the nail surface by a glass slide or a sharp instrument is recommended before applying medication. Painting with 2% gluteraldehyde solution (Cidex) is curative. There is no need to alkalinize this solution as reported.[14] There is also no need to worry about cross-sensitization to formaldehye.[15] (Gluteraldehyde will change the surface color of the nail plate to a tan color.) Other chemicals of similar nature will also effect a cure. Griseofulvin may be used systemically as well.

Treatment of Subungual Proximal Onychomycosis Due to Non-Dermatophytic Fungi

With the exception of Hendersonula toruloidea and scitalidium infection of the nails, avulsion of the infected nail plate will result in a cure. As yet, an antifungal agent that has successfully cured Hendersonula infection has not been reported. Miconazole, Pimaricin[16] or Thiabendazole may be tried.

Treatment of Dermatophytic Onychomycosis

The present treatment of choice is systemic Griseofulvin. It should be given until the nail is normal; thereafter, maintenance with a topically applied antifungal agent should be continued. The response varies remarkably between onychomycotic finger- and toe-nails.

Systemic Treatment

Treatment of Fingernail Onychomycosis (DSO, PSO)

Fingernail Onychomycosis has been thought to be exclusively produced by dermatophytic fungi. For practical purposes, this is true since the newly described nondermatophytic fungi (Hendersonula and Scytalidium) must be rare.

Griseofulvin will be curative if the dose and the schedules are not modified from what the original investigators[17] have described. A minimum of 1 g of microparticled, micronized or microcrystalline Griseofulvin should be used. Divided doses are preferred. A fatty meal continues to be important. This dosage *should not be reduced* even though the nail begins to improve. This is probably the most common error made by clinicians. Treatment should continue until the nail looks perfectly normal. Overtreatment rather than undertreatment is recommended since recurrences are likely with too little treatment. Treatment time for fingernails will vary to a maximum usually of 6 months (Fig. 52-53) To reduce treatment time with Griseofulvin, avulsion of the nail is definitely recommended (Fig. 54).

Polyethylene Glycol 4000—Griseofulvin

The latest of the improved Griseofulvin preparations recommends the use of half the dose of microsized Griseofulvin. This is based on improved gut, serum and tissue concentrations. As yet, there are no studies in onychomycosis, but in a well-controlled study on tinea pedis performed by the author the claims of 0.5 daily instead of 1 g microsized are confirmed. A minimum of 0.5 g should then be started and that dosage continued until the nail plate is completely cured and looks normal.

The data available on the cure rate of finger onychomycosis are scanty; however, the original observation of Blank and associates in 1959[18] remains true: in fingernails, approximately 90 percent (plus) cures can be achieved. Other investigators[19,20,21] have achieved lesser cure rates. A follow-up of these patients one year later showed that they remained cleared.[22]

Treatment of Toenail Onychomycosis (DSO, WSO, PSO, Candida Albicans Onychomycosis)

The result of treatment of toenail onychomycosis has always differed from that for fingernail onychomycosis in that it is always more disappointing. The reasons for this are not known. How the tropical shoe-clad environment effects a decreased cure rate is puzzling. The causative organism may also be nondermatophytic.

Dermatophytic onychomycosis. Naturally, systemic Griseofulvin should be used. A starting dose not less than 1 g microsized or 0.5 propylene glycol Griseofulvin daily should be given. If no improvement is seen in 1 month, the dosage should be increased (if the patient tolerates it).

The published cure rates are somewhat lower than the author's experience. Candida albicans and dermatophytic onychomycosis (mixed) had an incidence of about 4 percent.[11] Most of the patients seen by me are highly motivated to cure their onychomycosis. Fig. 54 summarizes well-controlled studies utilizing regular and microparticled Griseofulvin at various daily dosages. It also includes the effect of nail avulsion.

Historical experience with Griseofulvin in the treatment of toe onychomycosis.

(1) 1 g daily regular Griseofulvin: Hargreaves[20] cured 50 percent (8 out of 16) of the patients whom he treated for about 1 year; when he avulsed their nails, however, 82 percent (14 out of 17) patients were cured. Kaden[21] obtained 35 percent cure rates (29 out of 58 patients) when he avulsed the nail; his figures for nonavulsion are extremely low—10 percent. (2) 1.5 g. regular Griseofulvin daily: Russell and associates[19] cured only 35 percent of their patients (10 out of 32) after 1 year of treatment. Stevenson and Djavaniszwili[22] cured 42 percent of their patients and followed them after 1 year, finding them still cleared. (3) 0.5 g microxrystalline (microsized) Griseofulvin: Hagermark and associates[23] measured plasma levels of Griseofulvin using gas chromatography and, while treating their patients, found basically no statistical difference between serum levels. Only 40 percent of the patients (11 out of 27) were cured after nearly 2 years of treatment. They noted an initial improvement followed by a static effect of the disease in 60 percent of the patients. Of interest, although not statistically significant, is their remark that all those (40 percent) who were cured had mean blood levels higher than those who became static after an initial benefit.

Nondermatophytic onychomycosis. Because there is no reservoir and no propensity by the host to grow these organisms, simple avulsion is curative. The only exception is Hendersonula toruloidea. As stated above, this agent clinically can produce onychomycosis, tinea palmaris and tinea plantaris. Little information is available as to its sensitivities against the known antifungal agents, other than its resistance to Griseofulvin.[24]

Mixed onychomycosis. Mixed onychomycosis by yeasts and fungi is more common than suspected by the clinician. Unless all causal agents are identified, another failure will attributed to Griseofulvin.

Treatment of Candida Onychomycosis

Two clinical conditions are known to be produced by C. albicans. One is a type of white superficial onychomycosis which is seen almost exclusively in infants and very young children (similar to Fig. 10). This clinical syndrome is believed by some investigators to be self-healing. It has also been seen by the author and reported to be produced by T. tonsurans and M. canis. Most of the children seen by me had S.-linked ichthyosis, a *severe* atopic dermatitis or severe malnutrition, and one was mentally retarded. The treatment is application of an anticandidal antibiotic (Nystatin amphotericin B, Clotrimazole, Haloprogin, Miconazole, Econazole) topically. Avulsion is curative but, I believe, a rather severe method. Making the diagnosis is the most difficult problem. This syndrome is known in the Japanese literature[25] and not in the Western literature. It was brought to my attention by Dr. Lewis Capland at the University of Miami.

Candida albicans onychomycosis in children with chronic mucocutaneous candidiasis syndrome. The nails infected by C. albicans in these children are a foci from which the skin and mucosa are repopulated. The nails should all be avulsed at one sitting and anticandida antibiotic should be applied topically. Nystatin should also be administered orally until the nail plates look normal. I have maintained four children's skin cleared by this method. The syndrome may present with various clinical components, but usually the nail involvement is so classical that the clinician should be alerted. The coexistence of dermatophytic fungi has been reported and is not very unusual.

Topical Treatment

Topical Antifungal Therapy

Topical treatment for onychomycosis has been very discouraging. The primary reason is that very few, if any, antifungal agents penetrate the nail plate. Thiabendazole, a benzimidazole, demonstrates an excellent antifungal effect topically whenever it is applied in an alcoholic solution or as an ointment or cream under occlusion. In a polyethylene glycol base, however, it is much less effective. Proven at two university centers independently, it should be used under a rubber finger cot whenever the patient cannot tolerate Griseofulvin.[26] Attempts to add a transport chemical to penetrate the nail plate were successfully demonstrated[27-29]with Griseofulvin and dimethyl sulfoxide as a topical paint against onychomycosis. Recently, miconazole nitrate has been used in an alcohol solution for dermatophytic infections. Results are dramatic and therefore need further confirmation.[30] The solution is experimental.

General Considerations

After studying 400 patients with T. pedis and onychomycosis by sphygmography, Forck (in 1970)[31] found that their peripheral arterial blood circulation was considerably disturbed compared to normals. The reduction, according to the study, was one-half to two-thirds of normal.

Table I
Dermatophyte Fungi Reported to Produce Onychomycosis

Fungus	Geographical Area
Trichophyton rubrum	World-wide
T. mentagrophytes	Europe and America
T. violaceum	Europe, Africa, Near East
T. schoenleinii	Eastern Europe, North Africa, Near East
T. tonsurans	World-wide
T. megninii	Portugal and Spain
T. concentricum	Rarely reported (South Pacific, Guatemala, southern Mexico)
T. soudanense	Rare (Africa); not studied
T. gourvillii	Rare (Africa); not studied
Epidermophyton floccosum	World-wide
Microsporum gypseum	Uncommon (world-wide)
M. audounii	Rare (Europe, Africa, North America)
M. canis	Uncommon
M. persicolor	World-wide

Table II
Nondermatophytic Fungi Reported to be Etiologic Agents in Onychomycosis

Author & Year	Organism	Confirmed
Blomqvist[32] 1969	Arthroderma tuberculatum	No
Kaben,[33] 1962	Aspergillus candidus	Walshe & English,[34] 1966
Bereston & Keil,[35] 1941	A. flavus	Bereston & Waring,[36] 1946
Walshe & English,[34] 1966	A. fumigatus	Rosenthal et al.,[37] 1968
Bereston & Waring,[36] 1946	A. glausus	Walshe & English,[34] 1966
Bereston & Waring,[36] 1945	A. nidulans	No
Kaben,[33] 1962	A. sydowii	Walshe & English,[34] 1966; Zaias et al.,[38] 1969
Moore & Weiss,[39] 1948	A. terreus	Kaben,[3] 1962; Walshe & English,[34] 1966; Zaias,[42] 1966
Kaben,[33] 1962	A. ustus	Walshe & English,[34] 1966
Kaben,[33] 1962	A. versicolor	Walshe & English,[34] 1966
Negroni,[40] 1930	Cephalosporium species (many species since)	Walshe & English,[34] 1966; Zaias,[42] 1966
Rush-Munro et al.,[41] 1965	Fusarium oxysporum	Zaias,[42] 1966
Gip & Paldrok,[43] 1967	Phyllostictina sydowii	No
Brumpt,[44] 1949	Scopulariopsis brevicaulis	Very heavily confirmed; most recent review by Belsan & Fragner,[45] 1965
Gentles & Evans,[11] 1970	Hendersonula toruloidea	Campbell, 1940; Campbell et al.,[24] 1973; Eady & Moore,[47] 1974
Restrepo,[48] 1976	Lasiodiplodia theodromae	Not yet confirmed
Campbell & Mulder,[12] 1977	Scytalidium hyalinum	Peiris et al.,[50] 1979

Table III
Correlation of Direct Microscopic Examination for Fungal Elements and the Fungus Recovered From Nail Samples in the Absence of Dermatophytes*

	Negative	*Direct Microscopy* *Positive*	*Total*
Curvularia lunata	8	0	8
Penicillium citrinum	8	2	10
Aspergillus nidulans	7	2	9
A. sydowii	7	4	11
P. lilaceum	4	3	7
P. chrysogenum	3	1	4
Hormodendrum nigrecens	3	1	4
Arthroderma quadrifidum	3	3	6
H. cladosporidides	2	3	5
Scopulariopsis brevicaulis	3	5	8
Fusarium oxysporum	1	3	4
Cephalosporum oxysporum	1	4	5
C. acremonium	0	3	3
A. terricola	0	4	4
Aspergillus species	0	6	6

*Only one fungus recovered in all cases.

Table IV
Relationship of Yeasts Recovered and Demonstration of Fungal Pseudohyphae (KOH) in Toenails*

	No. of Nails *Isolated*	*Total* *KOH*	*KOH &* *Only One* *Organism* *Isolated*	*KOH &* *Other* *Organisms* *Isolated*	*KOH*
Candida albicans	21	12	5	7	9
Candida guillermondii	3	1	0	1	2
Candida parapsilosis	61	21	9	12	40

*Nails yielding other yeasts did not show pseudo-hyphae in direct microscopic examination (Candida intermedia, C. robusta, C. tropicalis, Torulopsis candida, T. glabrata, Trichosporum beigelii, T. capitatum, Rhodotorula mucilagenosa and R. rubra).

Table V
Superficial White Onychomycosis Causal Organisms

TOENAILS
Dermatophytes: Trichophyton mentagrophytes; almost all cases
Trichophyton rubrum; once reported?
Microsporum persicolor; often confused with T. mentagrophytes
Candida albicans; seen only in infants
Nondermatophytes: Caphalosporium s.p.s.
Aspergillus terrens
A. species
Fusarium oxysporum

FINGERNAILS
Very rare; mostly in infants with candida albicans
Trichophyton tonsurans

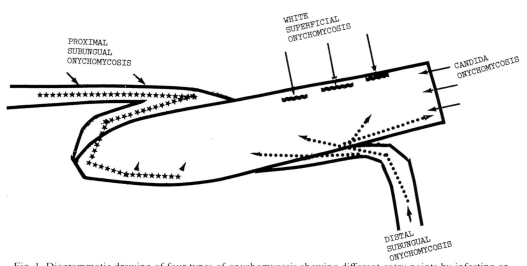

Fig. 1. Diagrammatic drawing of four types of onychomycosis showing different entry points by infecting organism.

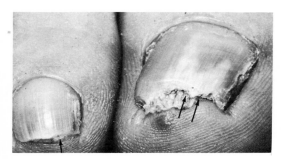

Fig. 2. Distal subungual onychomycosis (DSO), showing early invasion (arrow) to stratum corneum beneath nail plate; double arrow shows more advanced subungual debris by T. mentographytes.

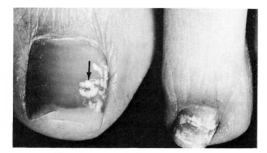

Fig. 3. White superficial onychomycosis. Arrow points to island of fungal involvement, T. mentagrophytes.

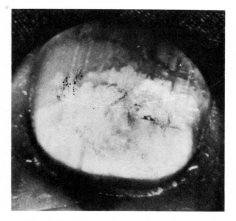

Fig. 4. Proximal subungual onychomycosis (PSO), showing involvement of nail plate proximally and subungually by T. rubrum.

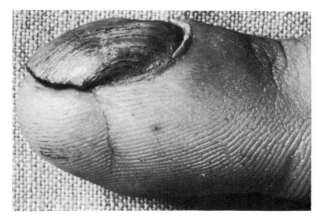

Fig. 5. Chronic mucocutaneous candidiasis. Candida onychomycosis nail plate.

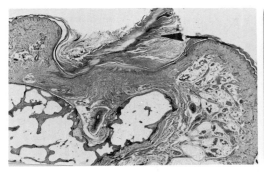

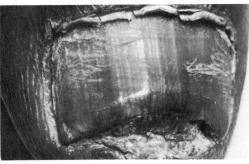

Fig. 6. Histologic section of distal subungual onychomycosis toenail. Arrow points to subungual debris mostly from nail bed and hyponychium. H&E X12.

Fig. 7. DSO, showing marked subungual involvement and fairly untouched nail plate. T. rubrum.

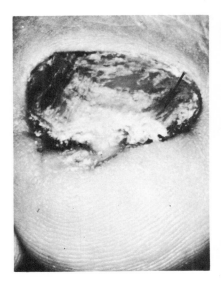

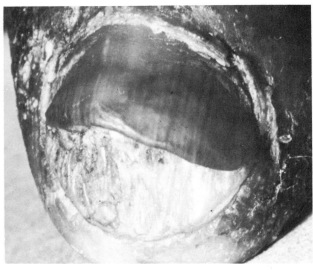

Fig. 8. DSO. T. tonsurans. Arrow points to "spriggy network" of Sowinsky and Alkewicz.

Fig. 9. DSO. Further involvement of nail bed with obvious uplifting of nail plate. T. rubrum.

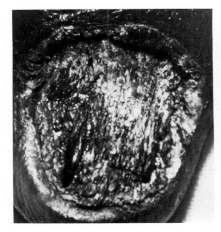

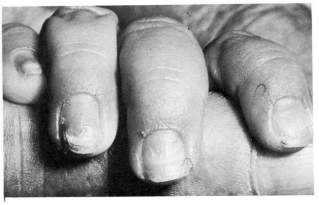

Fig. 10. DSO. Later stages, showing nail plate with marked nail bed hyperkeratosis. T. rubrum.

Fig. 11. Four-month infant, showing little finger and ring finger involvement of nail plate subungually and on surface by *microsporum gypsum*. Infant has sex-linked icthyosis.

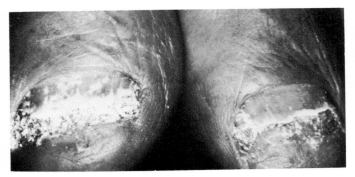

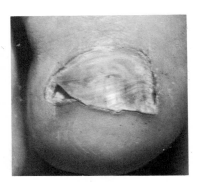

Fig. 12. DSO. Mixed infection, C. albicans and T. rubrum. Nail cut to show lysis.

Fig. 13. DSO. Cephalosporium.

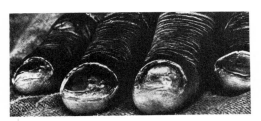

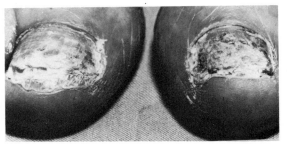

Fig. 14. DSO. Hendersonula toruloidea. (Campbell et al., *Br. J. Dermatol. 89,* 1973).

Fig. 15. DSO, T. rubrum, in patient with psoriasis (see Fig. 16).

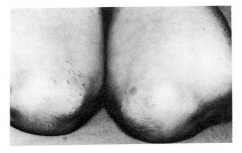

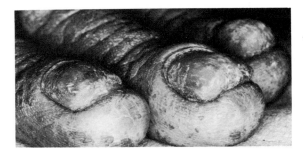

Fig. 16. Elbows of patient with psoriasis and onychomycosis (see Fig. 15). T. rubrum.

Fig. 17. Patient with Darier's disease. T. rubrum.

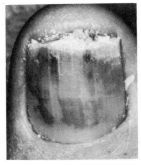

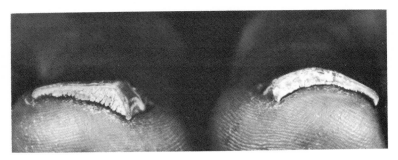

Fig. 18. Darier's disease with T. rubrum. Candida albicans and Pseudomonos.

Fig. 19. Lichen planus with T. rubrum.

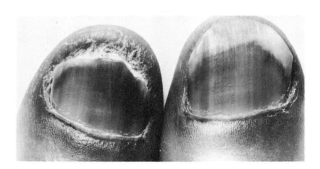

Fig. 20. Lichen planus with T. rubrum.

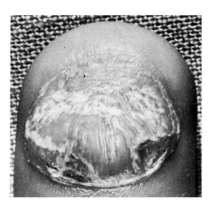

Fig. 21. Lichen planus with T. mentagrophytes.

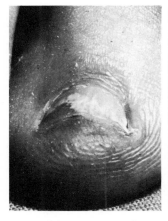

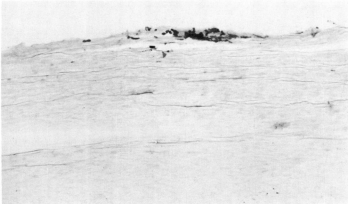

Fig. 22. White superficial onychomycosis (WSO). Fusarium oxysporum.

Fig. 23. Histologic section of WSO. Note fungal island on nail plate. PAS X120.

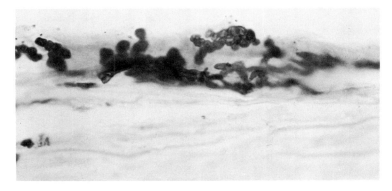

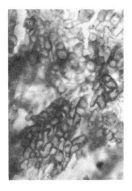

Fig. 24. Higher power of island in Fig. 23, showing fungus to consist of large, eroding bodies not typically seen in DSO but characteristic for this clinical disease. PAS X420.

Fig. 25. WSO. Large clusters of eroding bodies. Fusarium oxysporum *in vivo*. PAS X600.

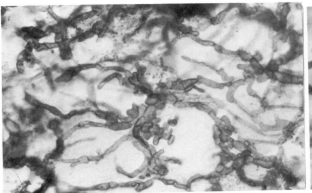

Fig. 26. WSO. Fusarium oxysporum hyphae, *in vivo* nail. PAS X400.

Fig. 27. WSO. *In vivo* nail with Cephalosporium species. PAS X420.

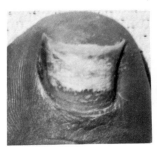

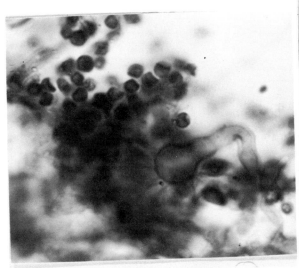

Fig. 28. WSO with Aspergillus terreus.

Fig. 29. WSO hyphae. *In vivo* nail from patient in Fig. 28, showing typical nonseptated hyphae of Aspergillus. PAS X420.

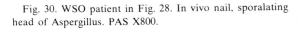

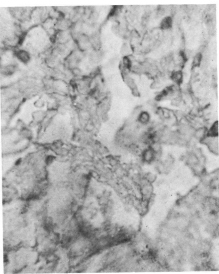

Fig. 30. WSO patient in Fig. 28. In vivo nail, sporalating head of Aspergillus. PAS X800.

Fig. 31. Patient in Fig. 30. Eroding bodies of *aspergillus terreus, in vivo* nail. PAS X640.

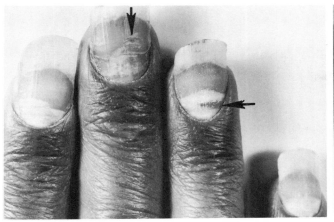

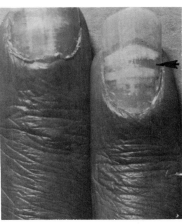

Fig. 32. Proximal subungual onychomycosis (PSO). Note involvement of nail with white area proximally. Fungus involves nail, periodically leaving normal areas (horizontal arrow).

Fig. 33. Patient in Fig. 32 approximately 2 months later, showing position of horizontal arrow now moving quite distally in finger.

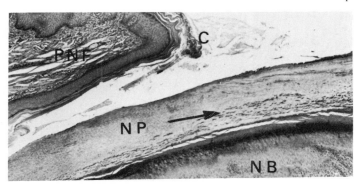

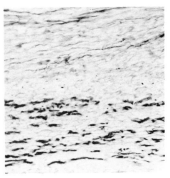

Fig. 34. Histologic section of patient in Fig. 32 through proximal nail fold, showing nail plate involved with fungus (arrow) at its ventral portion. PAS X120.

Fig. 35. Higher power (photomicrograph) of Fig. 34 (tip of arrow), showing detail of involvement of fungus at ventral portion of nail plate. PAS X120.

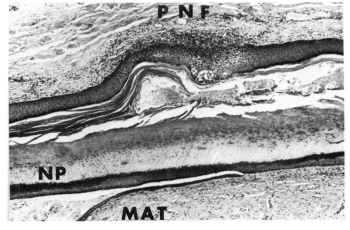

Fig. 36. Higher power of proximal nail fold area showing how fungus invades PNF stratum corneum and matrix area to involve nail through ventral portion. PAS X120.

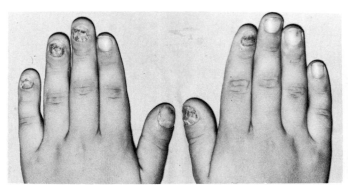

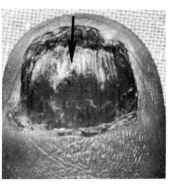

Fig. 37. Chronic mucocutaneous candidiasis onychomycosis (CMCO).

Fig. 38. Note involvement of nail throughout thickness (arrow down) by C. albicans.

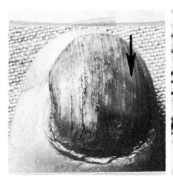

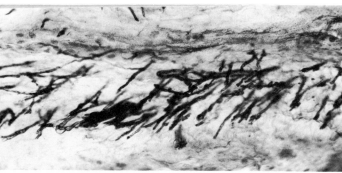

Fig. 39. CMCO, different patient. Thorough involvement of nail plate with C. albicans.

Fig. 40. Photomicrograph showing C. albicans. *In vivo* nails assume pseudo- hyphae which appear totally unlike elements of cutaneous candidiasis. PAS X240.

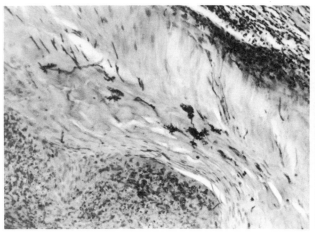

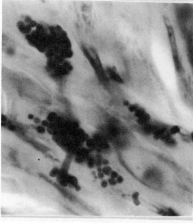

Fig. 41. CMCO, another area of nail plate of patient in Fig. 40, showing typical C. albicans configuration of organism PAS X120.

Fig. 42. CMCO. Higher power of Fig. 41, showing typical grape-clusters of fungus. PAS X1000.

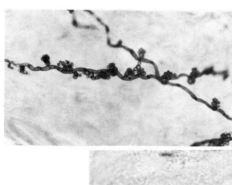

Fig. 43. CMCO. C. albicans in typical form, *in vivo* nails. PAS X120.

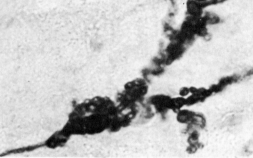

Fig. 44. CMCO. Eroding frond, C. albicans, *in vivo* nail. PAS X1000.

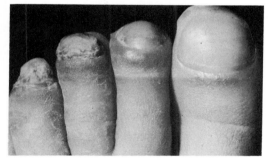

Fig. 45. Toes of mucocutaneous candidiasis patient showing bulbous fingertip and deteriorated nail plate.

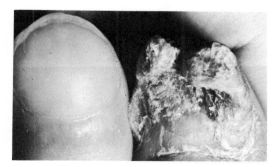

Fig. 46. Severely deteriorated nail plate typical of mucocutaneous candidiasis, Norwegian scabies and other cellular immunologic deficit states.

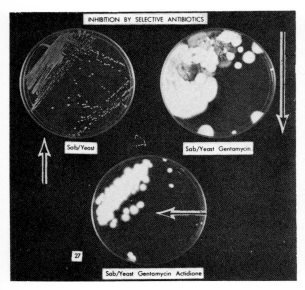

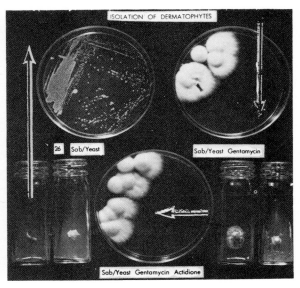

Fig. 47. Nail fungal recovery. Selection of proper culture medium is necessary. Patient #27 had bacterium grow (micrococcus) which produced antidermatophytic substance. This phenomenum could help explain positive direct examination and negative culture result. In nonselective medium, only bacteria grew (arrow up). In media with gentomycin, molds and dermatophytes grew (arrow down). In media with gentomycin and mold inhibitor Actidione, only dermatophytes grew (horizontal arrow).

Fig. 48. Patient #26 with onychomycosis. Same situation as patient #27 in Fig. 47.

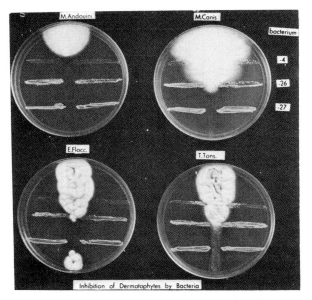

Fig. 49. Antidermatophytic action of various bacteria isolated from onychomycotic patients various bacteria (nos. 4, 26, 27) produce antifungal substances. Inhibition against M. Audouinii, M. canis, E. floccosum, and T. tonsurans. Inhibitions also exist against T. rubrum and T. mentogrophytes.

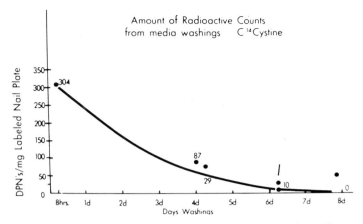

Fig. 50. Radiolabeled nail samples stabilize in media solutions. These samples are then used in testing.

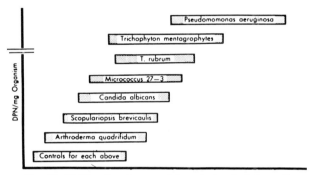

Fig. 51. Ability of various organisms to break down radiolabeled primate nail samples. Pseudomonas and T. mentagrophytes are best adapted. T. rubrum is poor nail destroyer and perhaps relies on other organisms inhabiting DSO niche for continuing nail invasion.

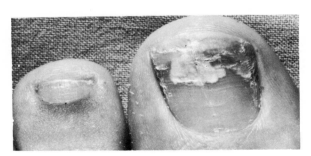

Fig. 52. Onychomycosis *T. Rubrum.*

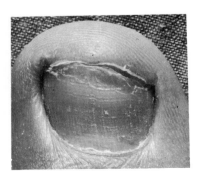

Fig. 53. Toenail in Fig. 52 treated with 1 g regular Griseofulvin for 6 months. Treatment should continue until toenail looks completely normal. Recurrences are likely if stopped too early, as shown here.

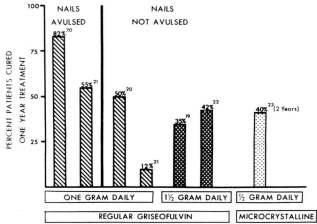

Fig. 54. Chart showing various Griseofulvin doses: 1 g, 1.5 g and 0.5 g daily of either regular or microcrystalline Griseofulvin with and without avulsion of nails. Treatment response of onychomycosis with various types of Griseofulvin and various doses. Small number on upper right of each column is reference. Abulsion is definitely an advantage.

NOTES

1. Zaias, N.: Onychomycosis. *Arch. Derm. 105*: 263-274, 1972.
2. Alkiewicz, J.: Transverse net in the diagnosis of onychomychosis. *Arch. Derm. Syph. 58*: 385, 1948.
3. Sowinski, W.: The "spriggy network." A new diagnostic symptom of onychotrichophytosis in vivo. Proceedings International Symposium of Medical Mycology, 1963, Warsaw, Poland. Edited by I.B. Rdzner and Marceli Stauber.
4. **Zapater, R. and Rudich, R.: Onicomicosis de Mano.** *Arch. Argentinos Dermatologia 19*: 3-4, 1969.
5. Jessner, M.: Über eine Neue form von Nagel Nagkosen (leukomychia trichophytica). *Arch. Derm. Syph. (Berlin) 141*: 1-8, 1922.
6. Reiss, F.: Leukonychia trichophytica caused by trichophyton rubrum. *Cutis 20*: 223-224, 1977.
7. English, M.P.: The saprophytic growth of keratinophylic fungi in keratin. *Sabouraudia 2*: 115-130, 1962.
8. Stümmer, A.: Subungual epidermophytic, trichophytic und favus. *Arch. Derm. Syph. (Berlin) 193*: 527-536, 1952.
9. Hanser, F.V., and Rothman, S.: Monilial granuloma. *Arch. Derm. Syph. 61*: 307-319, 1950.
10 Zaias, N., and Taplin, D.: An improved preparation for the diagnosis of mycologic disease. *Arch. Derm. 93*: 608, 1966.
11. Genles, J.C., and Evans, E.G.V.: Infection of the feet and nails with Hendersonula toruloidea. *Sabouraudia 8*: 72-75, 1970.
12. Campbell, C.K., and Mulder, J.L.: Skin and nails infection by Scytalidium hyalinum sp. Nov. *Sabouraudia 15*: 161-166, 1977.
13. Taplin, D., Zaias, N., Rebell, G., and Blank, H.: Isolation and recognition of dermatophytes on a new medium (DTM). *Arch. Derm. 96*: 203-209, 1969.
14. Suringa, D.W.R.: Treatment of superficial onychomycosis with topically applied gluteraldehyde. *Arch. Derm. 102*: 163-167, 1970.
15. Weaver, J.E., and Maibach, H.I.: Dose response relationships in allergic contact dermatitis: gluteraldehyde containing liquid fabric softener. *Contact Dermatitis 3*: 65-68, 1977.

16. Wildfeuer, A.: Die Wierkung von Pimaricin gegen Hendersonula toruloidea in Experimentellan Untersuchungen. *Arzeneimittal forschung (Drug Research) 22*: 101-104, 1972.

17. Hildick-Smith, G., Blank, H., and Sarkany, I.: *Fungus Diseases and Their Treatment.* Boston: Little, Brown, 1964, pp. 114-126.

18. Blank, H., Smith, J.G., Jr., Roth, F.J., Jr., and Zaias, N.: Griseofulvin for systemic treatment of dermatomycoses. *JAMA 171*: 2168-2174, 1959.

19. Russell, B., Frain-Bell, W., Stevenson, C.J., Riddell, R.W., Djavahiszwili, N., and Morrison, S.L.: Chronic ringworm infection of the skin and nails treated with Griseofulvin. *Lancet 1*: 1140-1147, 1960.

20. Hargreaves, G.K.: The treatment of onychomycosis with Griseofulvin. *Brit. J. Derm 72*: 358-364, 1960.

21. Kaden, R.: Klinische und mykologische Machuntersuchungen. Griseofulvin Behandelter Onychomykogen. *Mychopath. et Mycol. 25*: 351-360, 1965.

22. Stevenson, C.J., and Djavaniszwili, N.: Chronic ringworm of the nails. Long term treatment with Griseofulvin. *Lancet 1 (Feb. 18)*: 373-374, 1961.

23. Hagermark, O., Berlin, A., Wallin, I., and Boréus, L.: Plasma concentration of Griseofulvin in healthy volunteers and out-patients treated for onychomycosis. *Acta Dermatovener (Stockholm) 56*: 289-296, 1976.

24. Campbell, C.K., Kurwa, A., Abdel-Aziz, A.H.M., and Hodgson, C.: Fungal infection of skin and nails by Hendersonula toruloidea. *Br. J. Dermatol. 89*: 45-52, 1973.

25. Minomiya, S., Nabekura, K., Soh, Y., Doi, A., and Matsuda, Y.: Does infantile onychomycosis recover spontaneously? *Skin Research 10*: 655-659, 1968 (Japan).

26. Battistini, F., Zaias, N., Sierra, R., and Rebell, G.: Clinical anti-fungal activity of thiabendazole. *Arch. Derm. 109*: 695-699, 1973.

27. Macotela-Ruiz, E.: Personal communication, 1970.

28. Hiemisch, I.: Experiences with local administration of a DMSO incorporating antimycotic agent in onychomycosis. *Mykosen 13*: 175-177, 1970.

29. Kejda, J.: Nagelmykosen in der Praxis. *Castellania 2*: 251. 1974.

30. **Vanderdonckt, J., Lauwers, W., and Bockaert, J.: Miconazole alcoholic solution in the treatment of mycotic nail infections. *Mykosen 19*: 251-256, 1976.**

31. Forck, G.: Relationship between the blood circulation of the skin and the development of fungus disease. *Zental. Bakt. Parasitkde 212*: 544-553, 1970.

32. Blomqvist, K.: Arthroderma tuberculatum isolated from fingernail and beard. *Dermatologica 138*: 229-232, 1969.

33. Kaben, U.: Aspergillus candidus link als erreger einer Konychomykose. *Z. Haut Geschlechtskr. 32*: 50-53, 1962.

34. Walshe, M.M., and English, M.P.: Fungi in nails. *Brit. J. Derm. 78*: 198-207, 1960.

35. Bereston, E.S., and Keil, H.: Onychomycosis due to Aspergillus flavus. *Arch Derm. Syph. 44*: 420-425, 1941.

36. Bereston, E.S., and Waring, W.S.: Aspergillus infections of the nails. *Arch. Derm. Syph. 54*: 552-557, 1946.

37. Rosenthal, S.A., Stritzler, R., and Willafaue, J.: Onychomycosis caused by Aspergillus fumigatus. *Arch. Derm. 97*: 685-687, 1968.

38. Zaias, N., Oertel, I., and Elliott, D.F.: Fungi in toenails. *J. Invest. Derm. 53*: 140-142, 1969.

39. Moore, and Weiss, R.: Onychomycosis caused by Aspergillus terreus. *J. Invest. Derm. 11*: 215-223, 1948.

40. Negroni, P.: Una nueva mucedinacea parasita del hombre. *Rev. Soc. Argent. Biol. 6*: 653-663, 1930.

41. Rush-Munro, F.M., Black, H., and Dingley, J.M.: Onychomycosis caused by Fusarium oxysporum. *Aust. J. Derm. 12*: 18-29, 1971.

42. Zaias, N.: Superficial white onychomycosis. *Sabouraudia 5*: 99-103, 1966.

43. Gip, L., and Paldrok, H.: Onychomycosis caused by phyllostictina sydow. *Acta Derma Tovener 47*: 186-189, 1967.

44. Brumpt, E.: *Précis de Parasitiologie.* Paris: Masson, 1949.

45. Belsan, I., and Fragner, P.: Onychomykosen, hervorgerufen durch Scopulariopsis brevicaulis. *Hautarzt 16*: 258-264, 1965.

46. Campbell, C.K.: Studies on Hendersonula toruloidea isolated from human skin and nail. *Sabouradia 12*: 150-156, 1971.

47. Eady, R., and Moore, M.: Hendersonula toruloidea infection of skin and nails. *Trans. St. John's Hospital Derm. Soc. 60*: 104-108, 1974.

48. Restrepo, A., Arango, M., Herta, H., and Uribe, L.: The isolation of botryodiplodia theobromae from a nail lesion. *Sabouraudia 14*: 1-4, 1976.

49. Feurerman, E., Alteras, I., and Aruellyi, J.: The incidence of pathogenic fungi in psoriatic nails. *Castellania 4*: 195-196, 1976.

50. Peires, S., Moore, M.K., and Marten, R.H. Scytalidium hyalinum infection of skin. *Nails British J. Derm. 100*: 579, 1979.

CHAPTER 9

Darier-White Disease

Darier[1] and White[2,3] casually mentioned some nail abnormalities in their descriptions of the disease that bears their names. Half a century later, Ronchese[4] pioneered the concept that the clinical nail signs of Darier-White disease are unique.

CLINICO-PATHOLOGIC CORRELATIONS

The basic lesion is a papule and may occur in each component of the nail unit, i.e., the proximal nail fold, the matrix, the nail bed and the hyponychium, either singly or simultaneously. Depending on the extent and severity of the involvement (confluent papules) of these four components, the clinical signs range from inconspicuous to extensive alteration. Nail lesions usually eventually revert to normal but may persist for years.

The characteristic lesions are (a) distal, wedge-shaped, subungual striations (arrow up, Fig. 1; Fig. 2; double arrow, Fig. 3; index, Fig. 4; arrow, Fig. 6 (b) red, longitudinal, subungual striations (arrow down, Fig. 1; arrow, Fig. 3; index, Fig. 4; small arrow, Fig. 5; small arrow, Fig. 7), and (c) white, longitudinal, subungual striations (small arrow down, Fig. 1; index finger, Fig. 4; large arrow down, Fig. 5; large arrow down, Fig. 7). A less common finding is fragility and splintering of the nail plate, especially distally (Fig. 8). In severe cases, the nail plate was markedly thickened with massive, confluent, subungual keratoses (Figs. 8–12). These severe lesions were associated with dermatophytic fungi, Candida albicans or Pseudomonas aeruginosa, which modified the clinical picture (small arrow down, Fig. 1; index, Fig. 4; large arrow down, Fig. 5; large arrow down, Fig. 7) Patients suffering from superimposed onycholysis with C. albicans (arrow up, Fig. 8), or Pseudomonas present a varied clinical picture. Not all nails are characteristic of Darier-White, but usually one finger is involved only with the disease making the diagnosis available. Patients with onychomycosis as well as Darier-White do not present characteristic white-red lines and wedge dystrophy of the nail bed and hyponychium. One patient, *de-*

void of skin lesions, had nails with the characteristic clinical and histological features of Darier-White disease.

Nail Bed

White Longitudinal Streak—Subungual Keratosis

The most dramatic nail changes in Darier-White disease are in the nail bed, not in the nail plate. Depending on the number of epidermal ridges involved in the nail bed, either line lesions (white streak) (long arrow, Figs. 5, 7) or massive lesions (subungual wedge-shaped keratoses) (Figs 2, 3, 6) may develop.

In Darier-White disease, the nail bed epithelium is hyperplastic (nail bed line, Fig. 13; Fig. 14; double parted line, Fig. 15; Fig. 17 Figso Nail Bed). The nuclei may vary widely in shape and size (arrows, Figs. 17, 18, 19) and the cytoplasm is abundant and eosinophilic.

A remarkable finding is the presence of numerous multinucleate epithelial cells throughout the length and width of the nail bed. The multinucleate cells vary in number from binucleate to more than twenty nuclei in a cell (Figs. 21–24). The nuclei contain prominent nucleoli and well-defined nuclear membranes.

The histologic findings in the nail bed of Darier-White disease differ in three respects from those in skin: (1) absence of suprabasilar clefts, (2) presence of multinucleate epithelial giant cells, and (3) near absence of inflammatory infiltrate.

Red Longitudinal Streak

This common clinical sign of Darier-White disease represents an early lesion that, with time, develops into a white longitudinal streak.

Histopathologic examination of red streaks in nails of four patients showed (1) vasodilation in the subepithelial connective tissue of the matrix and nail bed, and (2) mild epithelial hyperplasia. Associated with the hyperplasia is minimal orthokeratosis and parakeratosis of the involved nail bed epithelium.

The white and red longitudinal streaks in Darier-White disease are a reflection of the unique relationship between nail bed epithelium and the subepithelial connective tissue: longitudinal, nearly parallel, epithelial ridges lock tongue-in-groove fashion, as do parallel dermal ridges (Fig. 21; Ch. I).

Matrix

In Darier-White disease, the nail matrix may be completely spared. When disease affects the matrix, its involvement is inevitably reflected in the nail plate as a white longitudinal streak.

In one biopsy, the white streak resulted from involvement of the distal matrix (lunula), where there were typical histologic changes of Darrier-White disease (Fig. 16). Focal epithelial hyperplasia of the matrix gave rise to persistent parakeratosis of the lower portion of the nail plate (double-headed arrow, Fig. 13), with resultant narrow linear leukonychia.

Involvement of only the proximal area of the matrix, with subsequent abnormality of the superficial portion of the nail plate, was rare.

Interesting findings in one specimen were multinucleated epithelial giant cells in the keratogenous zone of the matrix (Fig. 19). These unusual cells flattened as they ascended and were added to the nail plate.

Hyponychium

Hyponychial lesions consist of papules and plaques. The hyponychial epithelium is hyperplastic and the granular zone is thickened (arrow down, Fig. 13). Hyponychial cornified cells are wholly parakeratotic, containing large, hyperchromatic nuclei, some of them multinucleate.

Leukonychia Striata Longitudinalis

Leukonychia striata longitudinalis, described by Higashi[5], probably represents Darier-White disease.

Table I
Summary of Darier-White Lesions

Clinical Lesions	Site of Origin	Histopathologic Abnormalities
Red longitudinal subungual keratosis (early lesion)	Nail bed, often extending to hyponychium nychium and lunula	Mild epithelial hyperplasia with vasodilation
White longitudinal subungual streak (later lesion)	Nail bed, often extending to hyponychium and lunula	Epithelial hyperplasia with orthokeratosis and parakeratosis, subungual multinucleate epithelialgiant cells, epithelial giant cells, epithelial nuclear atypia
Wedge-shaped distal subungual	Distal nail bed and hyponychium	Epithelial hyperplasia with hyperkeratosis and parakeratosis
Splinter hemorrhages	Nail bed subepithelium	Hemorrhage around the blood vessels in the subepithelial longitudinal ridges
Proximal nail fold, flat keratotic papules	Proximal nail fold and volar epidermis	Papillary epidermal hyperplasia, orthokeratosis, suprabasilar clefting

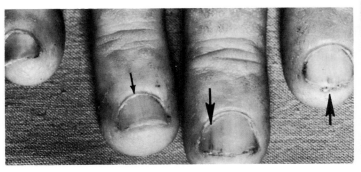

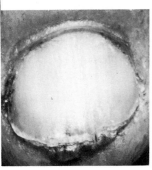

Fig. 1. Patient with typical Darier-White nail disease. Distal hyperkeratotic wedges (arrow up). Red (and white streaks small arrow down) that start from the lunula (large arrow down) end in hyponychium.

Fig. 2. Close-up of Fig. 1 (arrow up), showing hyperkeratotic subungual wedge. (Zaias & Ackerman, *Arch. Derm. 107*: 194, 1973, Fig. 3)

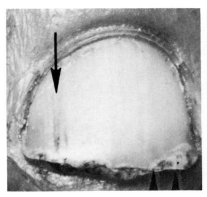

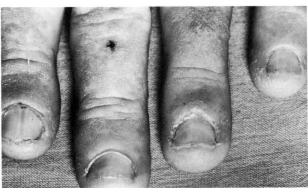

Fig. 3. Close-up of patient in Fig. 1 (large arrow down), showing red streaks typical of Darier's.

Fig. 4. Darier's of other hand of same patient showing similar changes. (Zaias & Ackerman, *Arch. Derm. 107*: 194, 1973, Fig. 6)

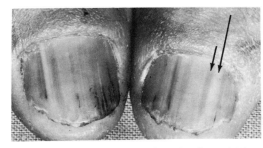

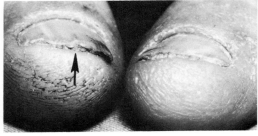

Fig. 5. Thumbs of same patient showing red (short arrow) and white (large arrow) streaks. (Zaias & Ackerman, *Arch. Derm. 107*: 194, 1973, Fig. 5)

Fig. 6. End view of thumbs of Darier's disease, arrow showing subungual hyperkeratosis.

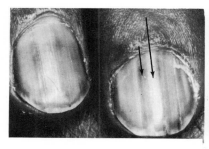

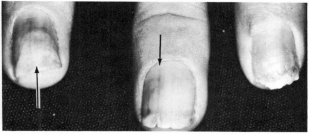

Fig. 7. White streaks (long arrow); red streaks (short arrow).

Fig. 8. Darier's disease—red streak (arrow down).

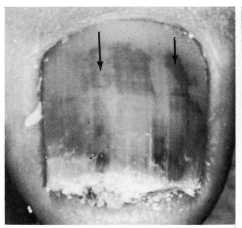

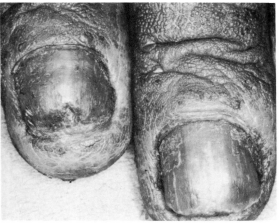

Fig. 9. Darier's disease, Candida albicans and Pseudomonas aeruginosa. Note onycholysis (arrows down) which clinically is very green.

Fig. 10. Darier's disease in patient with T. rubrum onychomycosis. Note thickened nails.

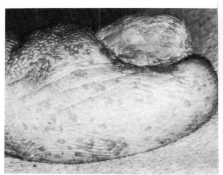

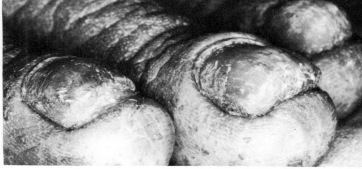

Fig. 11. Thickened nails of Darier's and T. rubrum. (Zaias & Ackerman, *Arch. Derm.* *107*: 195, 1973, Fig. 8)

Fig. 12. Darier's disease and T. rubrum. (Zaias & Ackerman, *Arch. Derm. 107*: 194, 1973, Fig. 4)

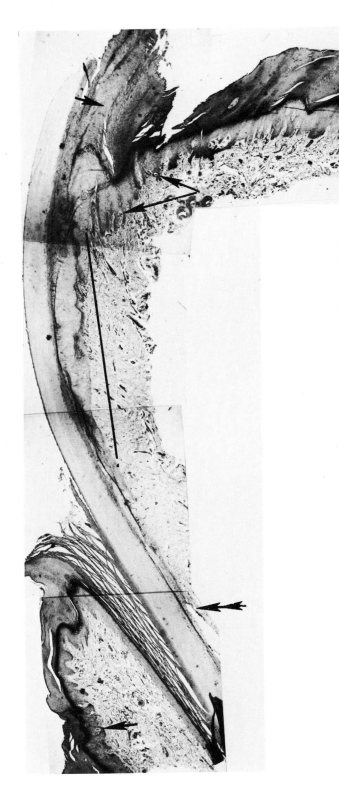

Fig. 13. Longitudinal photomicrograph of biopsy taken of patient in Fig. 12, showing entire matrix with typical artifact, suprabasilar cleft of Darier's (arrow up). Hyperplasia of nail bed (long line) and massive hyperkeratosis of the hyponychium (arrow down). Double arrow shows suprabasilar cleft typical of Darier's disease in hyponychium epidermis. H&E X50. (Zaias & Ackerman, *Arch. Derm. 107:* 195, 1973, Fig. 9)

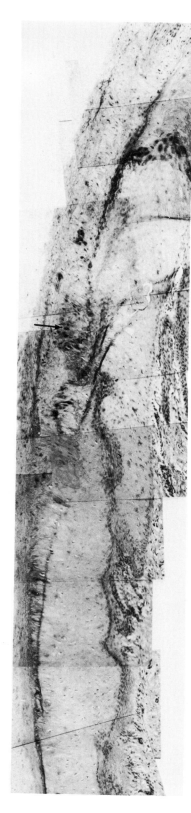

Fig. 14. Higher magnification of nail bed in Fig. 13 (line), showing hyperplastic epidermis of nail bed with resultant production of unusually large granular zone cells (arrow down) and confluent parakeratosis and hyperkeratosis. H&E X120. (Zaias & Ackerman, *Arch. Derm. 107:* 196, 1973. Fig 10)

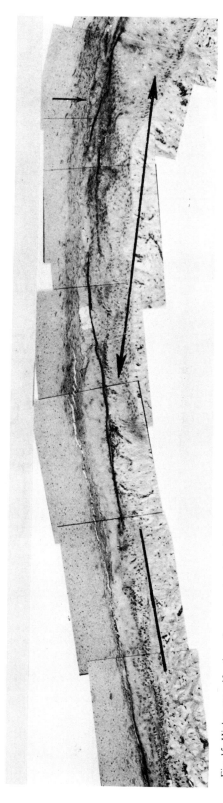

Fig. 15. Higher magnification of most proximal portion of nail bed in Fig. 13, showing that lesion is in fact linear plaque running length of various epidermal ridges of nail bed (double arrow). Note that nail bed epidermal hyperplasia begins near matrix (far left). H&E X120. (Zaias & Ackerman, *Arch. Derm. 107:* 196, 1973, Fig. 10)

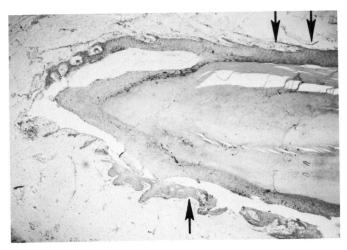

Fig. 16. Proximal nail fold and matrix area of patient in Fig. 13, showing suprabasilar separation of epidermis of matrix (single arrow up) and PNF (double arrow). H&E X120. (Zaias & Ackerman, *Arch. Derm. 107*: 198, 1973, Fig. 14)

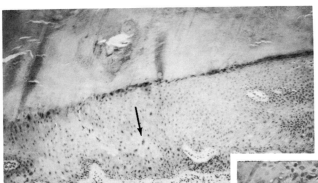

Fig. 17. Nail bed of another patient showing hyperplasia and atypia of cells in Malpighian layer (arrow down). H&E X240.

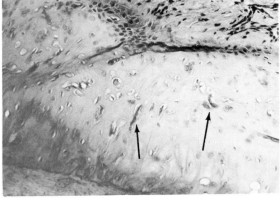

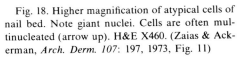

Fig. 18. Higher magnification of atypical cells of nail bed. Note giant nuclei. Cells are often multinucleated (arrow up). H&E X460. (Zaias & Ackerman, *Arch. Derm. 107*: 197, 1973, Fig. 11)

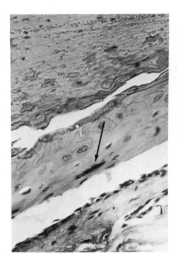

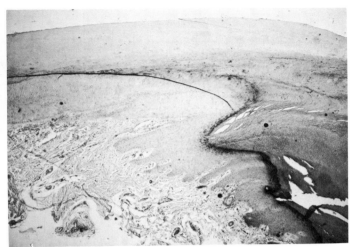

Fig. 19. Large nucleus of cell in lunula nail bed junction (arrow). H&E X900. (Zaias & Ackerman, *Arch. Derm. 107*: 198, 1973, Fig. 15)

Fig. 20. Photomicrograph of distal subungual keratotic wedge of horn, due to hyperplastic epidermis of hyponychium with massive dyskeratosis. H&E X120.

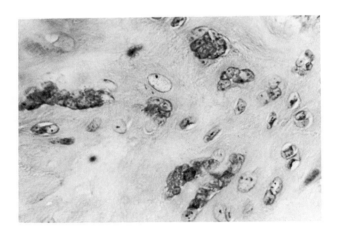

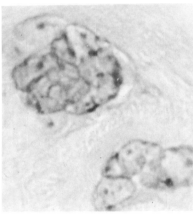

Fig. 21. High power of multinucleated large cells of nail bed only seen in Darier-White's disease. H&E X1000. (Zaias & Ackerman, *Arch. Derm. 107*: 197, 1973, Fig. 13)

Fig. 22. High magnification of multinucleated epithelial cells. H&E X2000.

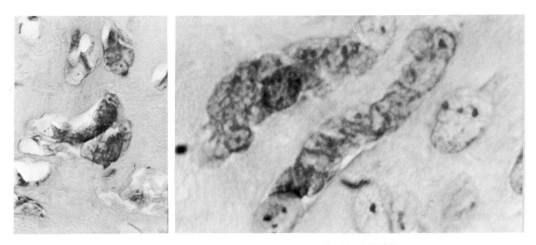

Fig. 23, 24. High magnification of multinucleated epithelial cells. H&E X2000.

NOTES

1. Darier, J.: Psorospermose folliculaire vegentate. *Ann. Derm. Syph. 10*: 592, 1889.
2. White, J.C.: A case of keratosis follicularis. *J. Cutan. Genitourin. Dis. 7*: 201-209, 1889.
3. White, J.C.: Keratosis follicularis, a second case. *J. Cutan. Genitourin. Dis. 8*: 13-20, 1890.
4. Ronchese, F.: The nail in Darier's disease. *Arch. Derm. 91*: 617-618, 1965.
5. Higashi, N.: Leukonychia striata longitudinalis. *Arch. Derm. 104*: 192-196, 1971.
6. Zaias, N., and Ackerman, A.B.: The nail in Darier-White disease. *Arch. Derm. 107*: 193-199, 1973.

CHAPTER 10

Lichen Planus

Nail involvement in lichen planus has been well documented. The reported incidence of involvement among patients with lichen planus varies considerably from less than 1 percent[1-3] to 10 percent.[4] The specific nail changes in lichen planus are not pathognomonic for the disease, as some of these can be identical with trauma of the nail. However, the diagnosis of lichen planus should be strongly considered when there are multiple nail lesions. Lichen planus of the nail without skin or mucous membrane involvement does occur.

Lichen planus nail involvement[5] may present as: (1) typical skin lesion with nail changes,[6] (2) atypical skin lesion, e.g., plantar ulceration of bullous lichen planus and nail changes,[7] (3) scalp lesion (alopecia) and nail changes,[8] (4) oral and nail lesions only,[9] and (5) nail changes only.[10]

The clinical appearance varies from slight roughening and ridging of the surface of the nail plate to total destruction and atrophy of the nail, depending on the location, severity and duration of the lesion.

Each of the nail unit constituents, singly or together, may be involved in lichen planus.

Interpretation of the clinical and the histopathologic specimens must take into account the dynamics of the nail plate formation and the variations in the size, shape and duration of the lichen planus lesion as it occurs in each nail constituent.

The pathologic process of lichen planus in the nail is essentially that seen in glabrous skin and hair. However, unlike the skin, the nail and hair may undergo a characteristic atrophy as the end result of the lichen planus inflammatory process (especially in the matrix). If the inflammatory response is severe, permanent atrophy may result, and alopecia or nail atrophy is clinically seen; with a milder inflammatory process, the clinical lesion may be only temporary.

MATRIX LESIONS

Longitudinal grooving and ridging of the surface of the nail plate (Figs. 1, 2, 5), first described by Dubreuihl[11] and termed "cannelures," may be a reversible nail plate change seen in minimally involved nails. This sign is the most common. The lesion results from temporary involvement of the most proximal areas of the nail matrix. If the process is short-lived, the furrows or longitudinal grooves disappear as the matrix repairs and normal plate is again produced. Samman[6] shows this well in Fig. 2. Similar changes have been described under the name "twenty nail dystrophy of childhood," but biopsies of two such cases proved to be lichen planus.

A variety of nail plate changes are seen according to the degree of matrix involvement and the scarring which results from the inflammatory process of the lichen planus.

A small lichen planus focus in the matrix may create an isolated island of scar which will show clinically as a bulge arising from under the proximal nail fold. The future nail plate will reflect this (arrow, Fig. 7, and less so, small finger, Fig. 8; Figure 9).

A severe inflammatory focus will result in destruction of the matrix and the adhesion of the overlying proximal nail fold epidermis to the nail bed epidermis. As a result, the nail plate in this area will never regrow and the adhesion is commonly known as a nail "pterigium." This process was first described by Friedman,[12] who termed it "Nivellierungsprozess" (arrow, Fig. 4). Often, partial loss of the matrix length can result in a thinner plate. If it is focal, the thinned nail plate will be flanked by nail plate of normal thickness (arrow, Fig. 4; thumb, Fig. 3; Fig. 10).

Complete involvement of the matrix and nail bed will produce a total loss of nail plate and permanent atrophy of the nail area (double arrow, Fig. 7; Fig. 14). A biopsy taken even as long as 6 months after the acute episode (arrow, Fig. 14) may reveal persistent histopathologic changes consistent with lichen planus (Figs. 15, 16).

NAIL BED AND HYPONYCHIUM LESIONS

Lichen planus papules involving the nail bed have been previously described.[11,12,13,14,15]

Distinct small[16] or linear[17] papules (Fig. 3) may be seen through the nail plate in the nail bed. These lesions disappear without any permanent damage (Figs. 6, 12). However, if the process is extensive and severe, the inflammatory reaction will result in a marked hyperkeratosis of the nail bed. Clinically, subungual keratosis and uplifting of the nail plate (arrow, Fig. 19; Fig. 20) is seen. In Negroes, postinflammatory subungual hyperpigmentation may also be seen (Fig. 19).

Any individual nail constituent (proximal nail fold, matrix, nail bed, or hyponychium) or any combination of these constituents may be involved at any one time with lichen planus.

UNUSUAL CLINICAL SIGN OF NAIL LICHEN PLANUS

In two children, ages 6 and 10, an unusual nail dystrophy was observed. The nail plate was absent, except in small areas where remnants could be seen (arrow, Fig. 17; Figs. 18, 21, 22, 23). There were no skin or mucous membrane lesions present, but one child did show small dime-sized scarring alopecic lesions in his scalp (Fig. 24). Repeated cultures for dermatophytes were negative. A biopsy of any involved finger (Figs. 25, 26) shows a normal proximal nail fold, while the matrix, nail bed and hyponychium were all involved with an-inflammatory reaction. Inflammatory cells hug the underside of the epidermis and form a sharp bandlike configuration. The classical histopathologic changes for lichen planus are seen (Fig. 26): (1) hyperkeratosis with hypergranulosis, (2) basal cell degeneration with incontinence melanin pigment, and (3) bandlike infiltrate consisting mainly of lymphocytes and histiocytes.

TREATMENT

The matrix lesion requires immediate treatment:

1. Locally, intralesional steroids (either by Dermojet or injectable), usually 3–5 mg/cc concentration; or

2. Systemically, prednisone, 20 mg daily for 2 weeks, then alternate-day treatment (Fig. 27) for children, 60 mgs for adults.

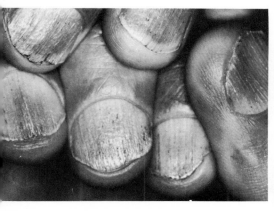

Fig. 1. Longitudinal ridging on all 10 nails seen in lichen planus and also in alopecia areata. This has been described as twenty nail dystrophy. Temporary.

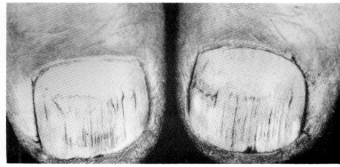

Fig. 2. Longitudinal striations are temporary in nature and regrowth of normal nail is seen after lichen planus has ceased to be active. (Samman *Brit. J. Derm 73*: 288, 1961. Fig. 1)

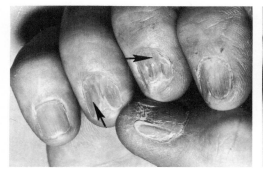

Fig. 3. Lichen planus, extensive papular lesions of nail bed (arrows).

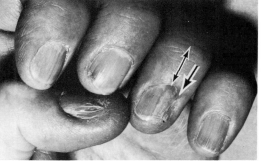

Fig. 4. Other hand of patient in Fig. 3, showing that lesion of lichen planus has focally atrophied matrix and proximal nail fold, resulting in pterigium (large arrow down) and red papule of lichen planus in the matrix (double arrow). (Zaias, *Arch. Derm. 101*: 265, 1970, Fig. 2)

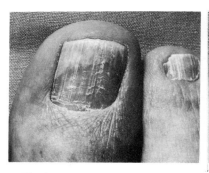

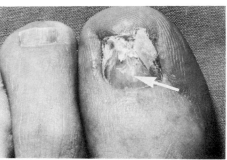

Fig. 5. Large toes of patient in Figs. 3 and 4, showing minimal changes of superficial portion of plate.

Fig. 6. Large toe of same patient showing past involvement of lichen planus with some clearing of the toenail (arrow).

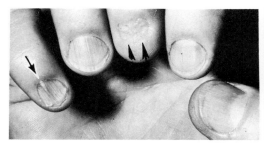

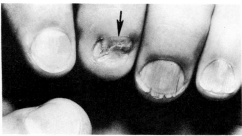

Fig. 7. Lichen planus in another patient involving more of matrix. Small papule of lunula produces split nail distally (arrow down). Middle finger totally destroyed. All components of nail unit have been scarred (double arrow). (Zaias, *Arch. Derm. 101*: 265, 1970, Fig. 4)

Fig. 8. Other hand of same patient showing remarkable symmetrical involvement of fingers as in previous hand, with partial destruction of matrix reducing its length and thus resulting in thinner nail plate, middle finger (arrow down). (Zaias, *Arch. Derm. 101*: 265, Fig. 3)

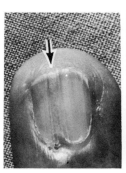

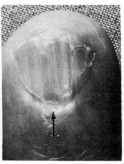

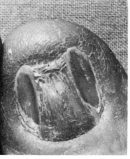

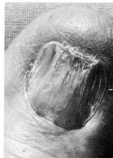

Fig. 9. Lichen planus lesion on another patient showing one small papule producing a longitudinal groove due to principle shown in Fig. 8. (Zaias, *Arch. Derm. 101*: 265, 1970, Fig. 1)

Fig. 10. Similar situation as in Fig. 9 in another patient. (Zaias, *Arch. Dem. 101*: 265, 1970, Fig. 1)

Fig. 11. Great toe of patient in Figs. 7 and 8. Larger papule of lichen planus has shortened matrix. Leaving abnormal center nail plate with two lateral normal pieces. Normally referred to as "angel wing nails."

Fig. 12. Minimal involvement of other toenail in same patient. Symmetrical lesion of counter foot.

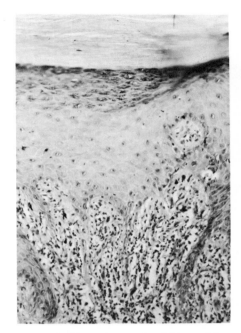

Fig. 13. Photomicrograph of biopsy taken from Fig. 7 (arrow down), showing proximal nail fold involvement with lichen planus. H&E X240. (Zaias, *Arch. Derm. 101*: 267, 1970, Fig. 13)

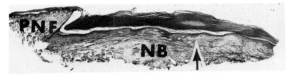

Fig. 15 Biopsy of area of arrow in Fig. 14, showing nail unit with very small focus of activity (arrow up). H&E X15. (Zaias, *Arch. Derm. 101*: 266, 1970, Fig. 7)

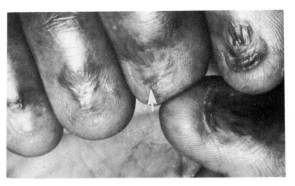

Fig. 14 Lichen planus affecting all fingers of hands with total destruction of all nail unit components. Red papule (arrow up) seems to be remaining active disease.

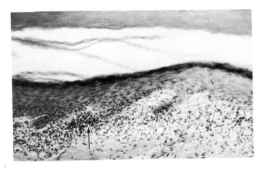

Fig. 16. Photomicrograph of area (arrow up) in Figs. 14 and 15, showing a small focus of lichen planus still active—typical hyperkeratosis, hypergranulosis, dermal-epidermal interphase activity, typical of lichen planus. H&E X120. (Zaias, *Arch. Derm. 101*: 266, 1970, Fig. 8)

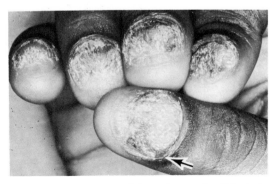

Fig. 17 Hypertrophic lichen planus of nail beds in child showing spicules of nail plate remaining (arrow).

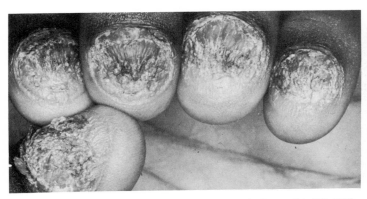

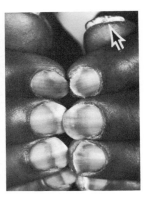

Fig. 18. Other hand of child in Fig. 17. (Zaias, *Arch. Derm. 101*: 269, 1970, Fig. 19)

Fig. 19. Hypertrophic lichen planus of hyponychium showing hyperkeratotic material under nail plate and pigmentation often seen in **lichen planus (arrow)**. (Zaias, *Arch. Derm. 101*: 267, 1970, Fig. 10)

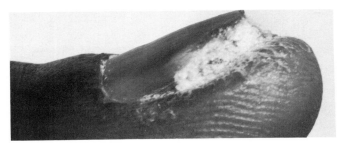

Fig. 20. Close-up of thumb showing hypertrophic lichen planus of hyponychium with massive hyperkeratosis subungually.

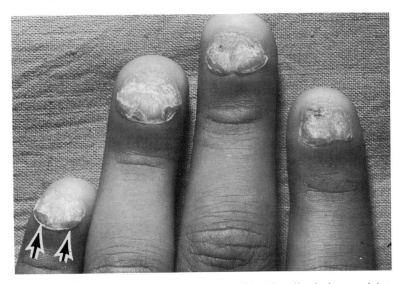

Fig. 21 Lichen planus in Caucasian boy, age 12, with nail spicules remaining (double arrow). (Zaias, *Arch. Derm. 101*: 268, 1970, Fig. 15)

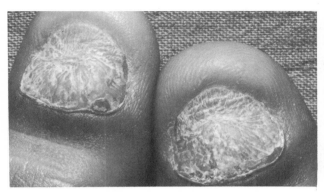

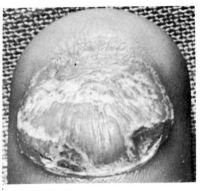

Fig. 22 Thumbs of same patient showing severe involvement of matrix with lamilations of nail plate rather than true nail plate.

Fig. 23 Finger, same patient, showing la-milations of nail plate. **Patient had coexi** tent Trichophytum rubrum infection. Nail plate may grow out normally.

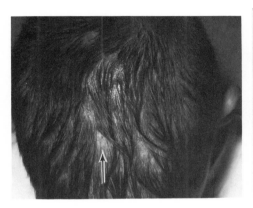

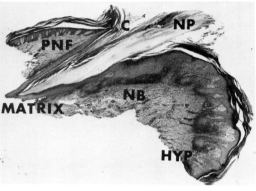

Fig. 24. Patient (Figs. 21, 22, and 23) also had **dime-sized alopecic areas of scalp. Graham-Little** syndrome. (Zaias, *Arch. Derm. 101:* 268, 1970, Fig. 16)

Fig. 25. Biopsy of patient in Fig. 23 through nail plate spicule showing proximal nail fold (PNF), matrix (M), nail bed (NB) and hyponychium (HYP)—typical lichen planus inflammatory pattern and other characteristics typical of lichen planus. H&E X12. (Zaias, *Arch. Derm. 101:* 268, 1970, Fig. 17)

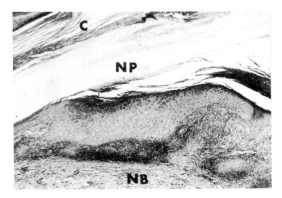

Fig. 26. Higher magnification of nail bed in Fig. 25, showing cuticle (C) nail plate overlying nail bed in-volved with severe lichenoid reaction and hyper-granulosis typical of lichen planus. H&E X240. Zaias, *Arch. Derm. 101:* 269, 1970. Fig. 18)

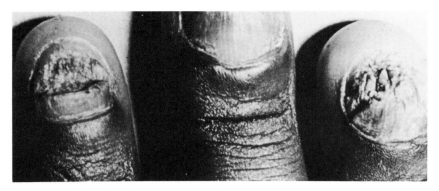

Fig. 27. New nail plate growth as response of prednisone 20 mg QOD for one month. Lichen planus.

NOTES

1. Little, E.G.: Lichen planus. *J. Cutan. Dis. 37*: 639, 1919.
2. White, C.J.: Lichen planus: a critical analysis of 64 cases. *J. Cutan. Dis. 37*: 671, 1919.
3. Heller, J.: Die krankheiten der Nagel, in Jadassohn, J.: *Handbuch der Haut-und Geschlechtskrankheiten,* Vol. 13. Berlin, Julius Springer, 1927, p. 222.
4. Samman, P.D.: Lichen planus: an analysis of 200 cases. *Trans. St. John Hosp. Derm. Soc. 46*: 36-38, 1961.
5. Cram, D.L., and Muller, S.A.: Unusual variations of lichen planus. *Mayo Clin. Proc. 41*: 677-688, 1966.
6. Samman, P.D.: The nails in lichen planus. *Brit. J. Derm. 73*: 288-292, 1961.
7. Gardner, R.K., Johnson, H.H., Jr., and Binkley, G.W.: Bullous lichen planus with onychatrophy. *Arch. Derm. 71*: 636-637, 1955.
8. Corsi, H.: Lichen planus associated with atrophy of nail matrix and hair follicles on scalp. *Brit. J. Derm. 49*: 376-384, 1937.
9. Gray, A.M.H.: Severe lichen planus of the mouth with loss of nails. *Proc. Roy. Soc. Med. 17*: 67, 1924.
10. Burgoon, C.F., Jr., and Kostrzewa, R.M.: Lichen planus limited to the nails. *Arch. Derm. 100*: 371, 1969.
11. Dubreuihl, W.: Lichen planus des ongles. *Ann. Derm. Syph. 2*: 606, 1901.
12. Friedman, M.: Nagelveranderungen bei lichen ruber. *Arch. Derm. Syph. 135*: 174-179, 1921.
13. Vero, F.: Lichen planus of the nail. *Arch. Derm. Syph. 26*: 677-683, 1932.
14. Sayer, A.: Generalized lichen planus with lesion of the palms and nails. *Arch. Derm. Syph. 41*: 813-814, 1940.
15. Zaias, N.: The nail in lichen planus. *Arch. Derm. 101*: 264-271, 1970.

CHAPTER 11

Psoriasiform Nail Unit States

Lack of facts about this group of diseases has resulted in the large number of clinical descriptions listed below. They have in common (1) a psoriasiform appearance and (2) a histopathological similarity. They differ in their clinical courses or their involvements with other organs and sites.

REITER'S SYNDROME

This entity can produce nail lesions (Fig. 1) which are indistinguishable from psoriasis. Other areas of involvement are the tongue (Fig. 2) and penis (Fig. 3).

PTYRIASIS RUBRA PILARIS (PRP)

The nails of PRP differ clinically from psoriasis in that they are always hypertrophic (Figs. 4, 5). Nail bed activity is moderate, with no great uplifting of the nail bed. The nail plate is thickened and ridged.

ACRODERMATITIS CONTINUA OF HALLOPEAU

This condition occurs around the fingers and toes. Though it is described as an entity, I have difficulty differentiating it from psoriasis (Fig. 6).

PARAKERATOSIS PUSTULOSA[1]

A clinical description consists of scaling, pustules, and venules around the fingers (thumbs and index) and toes, all occurring only in children. Histological proof making this a distinctive disease is not available. From my own reading, this "disease" includes contact dermatitis and psoriasis in children. Further proof is needed.

PSORIASIFORM ACRAL DERMATITIS

This could be a variant of psoriasis or keratoderma palmaris and plantaris (Figs. 7, 8). I have seen only one child with this disease and followed him to adolescence. The disease looks clinically like psoriasis but histologically is not. There is no epidermal rete elongation or confluent parakeratosis. There is, however, a leukocytic population involved.

SUBUNGUAL HYPERKERATOSIS

This clinical picture reminds one of psoriasis or lichen planus of the nail bed and hyponychium. Figs. 9, 10 and 11 show two patients who have this entity on most fingers and toes. This is permanent. In Figs. 12 and 13, one sees hyperkeratosis histologically: hypergranulosis without a lichenoid inflammatory reaction at the epidermal-dermal junction; no leukocytic psoriasiform reaction; no psoriasiform-like epidermal rete; with only occasionally focal Parakeratosis.

One patient constantly cleaned his nails (Fig. 9).

HYPONYCHIAL DERMATITIS

A patient who was a mechanic had fingers as noted in Fig. 14 for two years prior to seeing me. A contact dermatitis was suspected. He was patched to all solvents he worked with and the routine tray. All such studies were negative. Histopathologically, a great exudation of a serum-like material, also seen in other nail diseases, was the characteristic feature (Figs. 15, 16, 17). This material was PAS-positive (Fig. 17). The patient was lost to follow-up.

Acral Psoriasiform Reaction to Neoplasm

See discussion of Basex syndrome in Ch. 12.

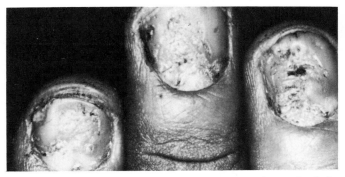

Fig. 1. Nail changes in a patient who has Reiter's syndrome. Psoriasiform nail changes with pits that can be confused with psoriasis.

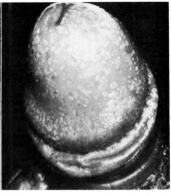

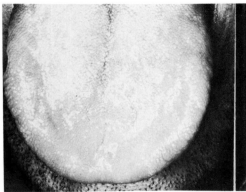

Fig. 2. Tongue of same patient with Reiter's syndrome.

Fig. 3. Penile papules typical of psoriasis and Reiter's syndrome.

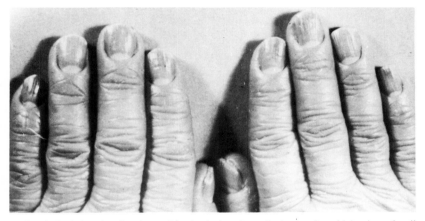

Fig. 4. Both hands of patient with pityriasis rubra pilaris showing thickening of nail beds and marked ridging of nail plate.

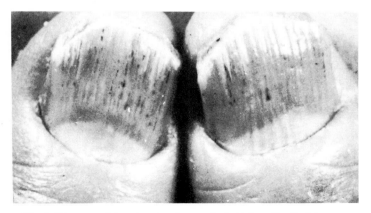

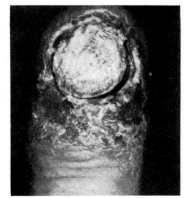

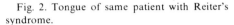

Fig. 5. Close-up of thumbs, showing marked ridging of nail plate—strongly suggestive diagnostic feature of pityriasis rubra pilaris.

Fig. 6. Patient with no history of psoriasis prior to developing, 3 months earlier, psoriasiform eruption on nail of one toe and of index finger. May represent psoriasis or acrodermatitis continua hallipeau.

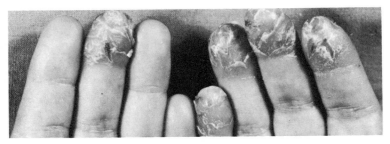

Fig. 7. Fingers of young boy with psoriasiform changes at fingertips. No other disease present. (University of Miami)

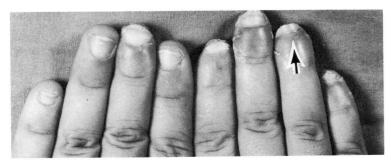

Fig. 8. Dorsal fingers of same patient showing short fingernail beds (arrow) on index and ring fingers of right hand. Biopsy was not typical of psoriasis. Undiagnosed (University of Miami).

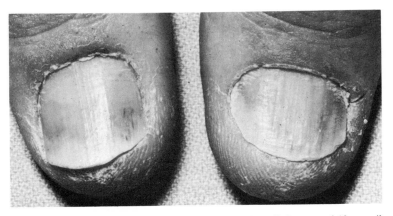

Fig. 9. An uncommon syndrome: the patient develops 10 finger- and 10 toenails that appear clinically to be involved with subungual hyperkeratoic process clinically looking very much like lichen planus; biopsy (Figs. 12, 13), however, does not correlate with this disease. Patient does not suffer from psoriasis elsewhere. (University of Miami)

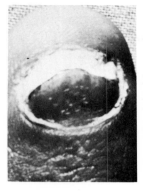

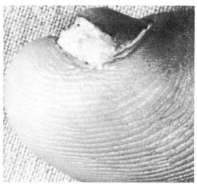

Fig. 10. Another patient with syndrome shown in Fig. 9.

Fig. 11. Subungual hyperkeratosis. Cross-lateral view of patient in Fig. 10.

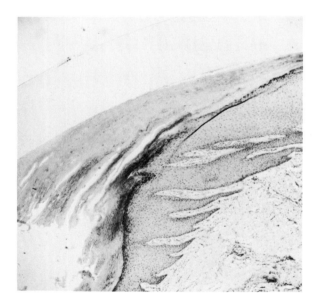

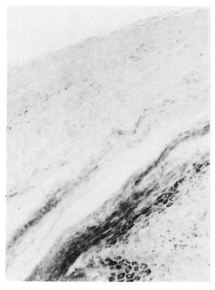

Fig. 12. Biopsy of patient showing massive subungual hyperkeratosis with focal parakeratosis, massive granular layer and almost no inflammatory response on the dermis. H&E X10 (University of Miami)

Fig. 13. Higher power of hyponychial area of Fig. 12, showing massive hypergranulosis and focal parakeratosis. H&E X100 (University of Miami)

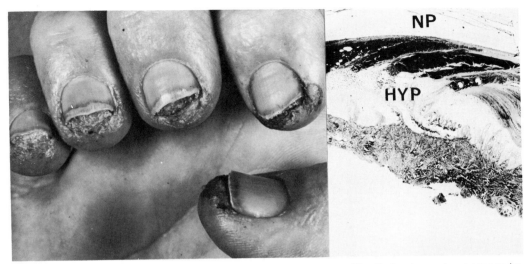

Fig. 14. Psoriasiform dermatitis involving fingertips, hypony-chium and distal nail bed of white male with unusual history and histopathology.

Fig. 15. Involvement restricted to hy-ponychium and production of exudative serum-like material. PAS X20. (Univer-sity of Miami)

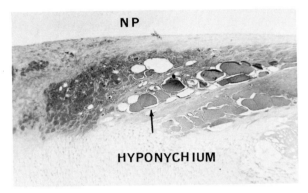

Fig. 16. Higher power of area in Fig. 15, showing serum-like material arising from epidermis and depositing among horny hyperkeratosis. H&E X240. (University of Miami)

NOTES

1. Hjorth, N., and Thomsen, K.: Parakeratosis pustulosa. *Brit. J. Derm.* 79: 527-532, 1967.

CHAPTER 12

Hair and Nails

Hair and nails differ in their specific biochemistry and anatomy. Yet, in spite of the overt differences, they must have evolved from a common structure. Just for fun, imagine a hair to be a nail unit rolled up into a cylindrical form with the nail plate in the center of the tube. There is anatomical similarity between them; i.e., the internal root sheath epidermis of the hair is analogous to the nail bed epidermis. They share diseases that affect them similarly. Take, for instance, alopecia areata: this disease produces the well-known temporary patch of local hair loss and also results in temporary nail plate lesions. Lichen planus affecting the hair results in permanent atrophy, as is the case with the nail matrix.[6]

ALOPECIA AREATA

The typical changes noted on the nail unit are restricted to the proximal matrix and result in the production of pits on the surface of the nail plate. The pits are shallower than in psoriasis and tend to have a geometric arrangement. This pattern has been called "Grid," "Screen," etc. (Figs. 1, 2, 3). These pits are temporary. Approximately two-thirds of all patients with alopecia areata have nail changes.[1]

Little is known about the exact relationship between the alopecic area and the nail changes.

ALOPECIA UNIVERSALIS, TOTAL VITILIGO, AND NAIL CHANGES

This interesting syndrome was first written up by Lerner.[2] Healthy patients undergo a series of events starting with diffuse alopecia (black hairs falling out first), leading to alopecia universalis, total vitiligo, and finally showing roughening of the superficial nail plate surface, nail plate brittleness and softening. Although the alopecia is permanent, the nail plate changes seen in this syndrome may be reversible.[3] Steroids are of questionable efficacy for the alopecia, but they may be of help for the onychodystrophy.

CONGENITAL ALOPECIA, ONYCHODYSTROPHY AND PALMAR-PLANTAR KERATODERMA

Sierra and Mesa[4] reported on a family of seventeen who presented nine members with alopecia universalis (some with no hair follicles, some with hypotricosis), onychodystrophy and keratoderma. There were other ectodermal abnormalities involving sebaceous and eccrine glands, and opthalmic as well as nervous system and mesodermal abnormalities.

BRITTLE NAILS IN AMINOGENIC ALOPECIA (ARGININOSUCCINIC ACIDURIA)

This rare condition, reported by Shelly and Rawnsley,[5] presented brittle nails after the hair began to fall out.

LICHEN PLANUS

Lichen planus is another disease where permanent alopecia and permanent nail dystrophy can co-occur. (See Chapter X.)

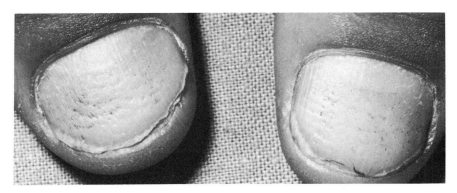

Fig. 1. Thumbs of patient with alopecia areata showing very fine stipling resembling grid pattern seen on surface of nail. (University of Miami)

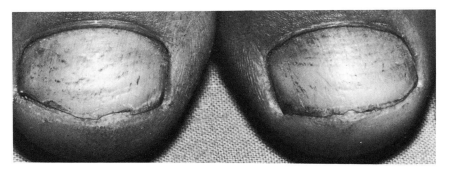

Fig. 2. Toenails of same patient showing changes similar to those in Fig. 1. (University of Miami)

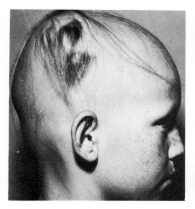
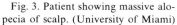
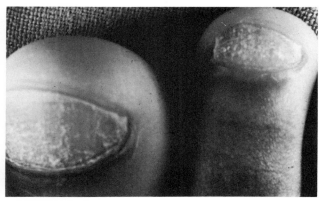

Fig. 3. Patient showing massive alopecia of scalp. (University of Miami)

Fig. 4. Fine sandpaper appearance of youngster's fingernails with
congenital ectodermal defect and alopecia. (University of Miami)

NOTES

1. Klingmuller, G., and Reeh, E.: Nagelgrubchen und deren Familiare Haufungen Dei Der Alopecia Areata. *Arch. Klin. Exp. Dermat. 201*: 574-581, 1955.
2. Lerner, A.B.: Three unusual pigmentary syndrome. *Arch. Derm. 83*: 17-105, 1961.
3. Demis, J.D., and Weiner, M.A.: Alopecia universatis, onychodystrophy and total vitiligo. *Arch. Derm. 88*: 195-201, 1963.
4. Sierra, H.G., and Mesa, J.C.: Alopecia, distrofia ungueal y queratodermia palmoplantar congenitas. *Medicina Cutanea Year II*: 369-372, 1968.
5. Shelley, W.B., and Rawnsley, H.M.: A minogenic alopecia, look of hair associated with arginino succinic aciduria. *Lancet* 1327-1328, 1965.
6. Zaias, N.: The nail in lichen planus. *Arch. Derm. 101*: 264-271, 1970.

CHAPTER 13

Paronychia

The "inflammation," redness and swelling of the lateral and/or proximal nail fold is known as paronychia. Usually, on a clinical basis, two types can be diagnosed:

1. Acute paronychia—symptoms and signs occurring acutely
2. Chronic paronychia—insidious chronic development of signs and symptoms

ACUTE PARONYCHIA

This clinical syndrome is attributable to the formation of an abcess or cellulitis by a microbiologic agent (see Table I), most commonly staphylococcus aureus. The introduction of the causal agent into the proximal nail fold rapidly results in redness, swelling and pain leading to an abcess or cellulitis. It usually follows a history of trauma or recent hangnail in the proximal nail fold. Diagnosis of the causal agent and specific treatment consistently result in a cure. Incision and drainage, when applicable, should be performed (Figs. 1, 2).

Material for culture must come from the depth of the abcess or cellulites. Sterilization of the surface of the skin is mandatory or false causal agents will be cultured (70% ethyl alcohol swabbed for 2 to 5 minutes or any iodine solution will suffice).

Acute paronychia is not a precursor of chronic paronychia. Acute paronychia has been described to occur by staphylococcus aureus, streptococcus pyogenes, gram-negative bacteria like eikenella,[1] veilonella,[2] herpes simplex[3] and many unreported organisms.

CHRONIC PARONYCHIA

In contrast with acute paronychia, chronic paronychia is an insidious process which often goes unnoticed by the patient. The exact time of onset may be vaguely remembered. Redness and mild swelling of the PNF, and related to any overt trauma, is the earliest sign. The process starts with either the lateral or the proximal nail fold as a focus. With increasing swelling of this area, there appears to be a space formed between the PNF and the nail plate. The cuticle or horny layer of the PNF is absent; in its place, coarse scaling or none may occur. The process then moves to all areas of the lateral and proximal nail folds. If swelling and redness are severe, nail folds show buttresses, commonly known as "bolster swellings," and the newly created space enlarges (Figs. 3, 4, 5).

A thin cheeselike material often can be expressed from the depths of the now-formed proximal nail groove. The patient can show this by a milking action from proximally to distally. More will be said about this "pus." The clinical disease may now be months old, and the patient may experience an acute onset of further redness, swelling and severe pain in one particular area of the PNF. This usually brings the patient to seek medical advice, the main concern, aside from the severe pain, being that an abundance of more liquid pus is coming out which might spread the infection throughout. This is never the case. The acute flare is due to a secondary bacterial infection which is short-lived—usually 7 to 10 days. These little abcesses or cellulitic foci drain into the depth of the PN groove and are self-healing. Depending on the hand-oriented habits of the patient, these acute attacks may be very frequently experienced (usually in a very waterborne environment, i.e., laundering, etc.). Occasionally, other artifacts, such as wax,[5] can become lodged in the PNF. If the patient seeks medical advice, the unsuspecting physician will treat it with systemic antibiotics and local measures, claiming a therapeutic success. After the acute flare ends, the clinical course is the same as it was previously.[4]

With increasing damage to the more proximal areas of the PNF, those near the proximal matrix, the nail plate will emerge with typical transverse grooving leading to matrix damage. There are a series of transverse grooves on the nail plate which are interspaced among normal nail plate and are transient. Permanent damage can occur, since the patient may have the identical clinical picture for 12 years (Fig. 5).

Histology

Few accounts are available by which to reconstruct the histopathology of paronychia. My own plus Stone's[6] biopsises showed minimal or variable epidermal involvement (spongiosis, parakeratosis). The dermal infiltration consists primarily of lymphohistocytic and numerous plasma cells. Marked edema and vasodilations are present. The cuticle shows hyphae of Candida albicans.

Microbiology

The amazing fact about chronic paronychia is that the yeast Candida albicans can be recovered from a very typical lesion in a very high incidence (over 80% of the time). The question we all ask is: What is the role of Candida albicans in the production of chronic paronychia?[7] Since all agree that the water-borne environment is the right ecologic environment for candida albicans to flourish, we can assume that C. albicans is secondary to the water-borne environment. Various factors are known:

1. Whittle,[8] Ganor[9] and others have attempted to produce chronic paronychia clinically by application of C. albicans, but all have failed. Stone,[7] on the other hand, has claimed success. The clinical picture produced was very minimally that of chronic paronychia.

2. If C. albicans were the primary causal factor in chronic paronychia,[11] treatment with anti-candidal medications would terminate the disease process in a pattern befitting a

microbiologic disease. This, however, is not the case. Although there are reports of cures of chronic paronychia and onychias with Pimaricin[12] and other drugs, it takes a very long time (months rather than weeks) for cures to occur. This is not in favor of C. albicans playing a significant primary role.

Many papers have been written about the association of Candida albicans and chronic paronychia, particularly as to the source of the yeast that settles in the PNF. Ganor[9] showed in Israeli women that the mouth and the rectum had a higher prevalence of C. albicans than did the vagina of patients with chronic paronychia.

Incidence

It is a fact that chronic paronychia affects the young female predominately[13] the various reports available agree that the peak age groups are from 20 to 40. What can women of this age do to be rewarded so miserably? Most logically, it is thought that the water-borne environment surrounding all chores of the child and home is incriminated. This age span is also the peak age of colonization of Candida albicans in their stool, vagina and mouth. Both of these factors are again common in the infants and young children which they may be handling.

Experimental Data

Chronic paronychia has been reported to occur in a higher incidence among diabetics as compared to nondiabetic controls.[13]

In children[14] and rhesus monkeys[15] who suck their thumbs, a lesion which is clinically identical to chronic paronychia has been reported. C. albicans was present in all cases.

Summary

This perplexing syndrome, seen mostly in females of a specific age group (20 to 40) who are influenced by a waterborne environment and who also harbor Candida albicans as a permanent resident of their PN groove flora, appears to have no satisfactory etiologic theory to explain all the facts of the clinical syndrome.

Treatment

In some cases, the most rewarding instructions one can give the patient is that he take a vacation or stop his present occupation. The water-borne environment is what is usually discontinued by such a suggestion. In men with chronic paronychia, this is certainly very true. It almost always occurs in bartenders, janitors, fruit juicers, strawberry pickers, etc. Among women, only a percent of patients will improve and usually these are patients who know this will be the case if they discontinue wetting their hands.

The next most useful instruction is to warn the patient against wearing rubber gloves, as any occlusion will result in a continuation of the disease. I myself have retrieved C. albicans from gloves and do not recommend them. The patient dries her hands and uses whatever treatment has been prescribed.

Topical steroid preparations, as ointments, have performed best for me. If Candida is present, one must *add* an anti-Candida antifungal agent. Today, there are many to choose from e.g., Polyene antibiotics, Miconazole, Clotrimazole, Haloprogin, and more new ones coming. Personally, I use Nystatin powder. Systemic corticosteroids, prednisone 60 mg q.d. 4–5 days, will obliterate the clinical picture for as long as the patient takes the steroid. I have used this prior to important social events that patients need to attend. The patient needs 1 week of treatment before the fingers will look normal. If the patient has had her disease for many years, it is less likely to normalize.

Typical anti-Candida preparations (above) do not work. The "seal" technique (nail polish to the PNF) works, in my hands, in fewer rather than in most patients.

Discussion

My own views on this subject reflect a disappointment with the primary etiology by Candida albicans. I believe that the barrier of the PNF, specifically its ventral, thinner component, becomes damaged, making the entrance to the living epidermis easier for a cvaried number of possible chemical agents which ultimately result in the clinical syndrome of chronic paronychia. The water-borne environment facilitates the penetrability of these chemicals directly or indirectly (promoting a colonization of C. albicans which will then break down the barrier). By what mechanism a chemical results in chronic paronychia is difficult to state clearly. It is also true that chronic paronychia existed years before our modern chemicals related to the household came into play with the housewife, the major victim of chronic paronychia.

Therefore, I theorize that a chemical originating from many sources, but mainly from vegetable origin, repeatedly contacts the PNF: and when the PNF epidermal barrier is sufficiently damaged, it sets up a sequence of events which will end up as chronic paronychia. Immediate contact hypersensitivity,[16,17] recently popularized, has helped me to consolidate my theory. Contact with everyday foodstuffs has now been reported to produce clinical lesions such as edema, redness, urticarial wheels and vesiculations. These compounds usually need to have access through the epidermal barrier; thus, in proving them etiologic agents, a scratch test is required (if using normal skin) rather than epicutaneous patch testing. The list of these foods (compounds unknown) is becoming extensive. They include flour, turkey skin, ground lamb, potatoes, fish, shell fish, cheese, endive, chicory and lettuce. In addition, the histology of such reactons is strikingly similar to that of chronic paronychia.[17]

The role of delayed hypersensitivity also contributes to the clinical picture. Delayed contact hypersensitivity to vegetable matter is voluminous.[18-20] These foodstuffs are listed in Table I. New prospective chefs may be patch-tested to food listed in Table II. The therapeutic responses of steroids, either topical or systemic, overshadow the therapeutic response to any microbiologic agents or the avoidance of the water-borne environment. Therefore, chronic paronychia could result from simultaneous or separate occurrences of immediate and delayed hypersensitivities to chemicals in everyday food items.

Table I
Foodstuffs Positive Patch-tested in 53 Patients With Hand Eczema[18]

Garlic
Onion
Tomato
Carrot
Hisbiscus Esculentus (okar, lady fingers, kimbombo)
Ginger root
Solanium malongena (Malanga, Brinjal)
Radish
Cauliflower
Potato
Gourd (Cucuberta maxima)
Cucumber
Bean
Turnip
Coriander
Smooth luffa
Spinach

Table II
Foodstuffs Found Allergic in Food Handlers[20]

Onion
Garlic
Chives
Leek
Carrot
Cucumber
Horseradish
Lemon Peel
Endive
Lettuce
Asparagus
Artichoke

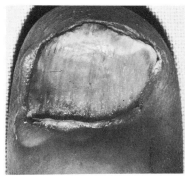

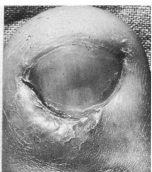

Fig. 1. Acute paronychia, staphylococcus aureus. Secondary to hangnail. (University of Miami)

Fig. 2. Acute transient (no bacteria recovered) paronychia.

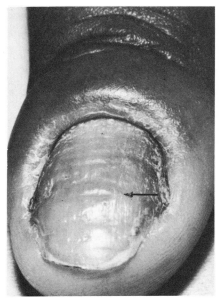

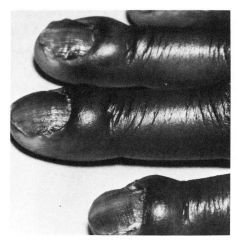

Fig. 3. Chronic paronychia, three months, in male janitor. (University of Miami)

Fig. 4. Note PNF edematous. (University of Miami)

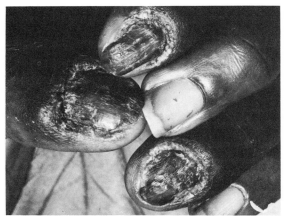

Fig. 5 Chronic paronychia with permanent changes, now twelve years old. (University of Miami)

NOTES

1. Barton, L.L., and Anderson, L.E.: Paronychia caused by HB-1 organisms (Eikenella corrodeus). *J. Pediatrics 21*: 372-373, 1972.

2. Sinniah, D., Sandiford, B.R., and Dugdale, A.E.: Subungual infections of the new born, an institutional outbreak of unknown etiology, possibly due to Veillonella. *Clin. Pediatrics 11*: 690-692, 1972.

3. Muller, S.A., and Herrmann, E.C.: Association of stomatitis and paronychias due to herpes simplex. *Arch. Derm. 101*: 396-402, 1970.

4. Stone, O.J., and Mullins, J.F.: Chronic paronychia, clinical aspects and therapy. *Clin. Med. 73*: 31-34, 1966.

5. Stone, O.J., Mullins, J.F., and Head, E.S.: Chronic paronychia, occupational material. *Arch. Environmental Health 9*: 585-588, 1964.

6. Stone, O.J., and Mullins, J.F.: Chronic paronychia, microbiology and histopathology. *Arch. Derm. 86*: 114-117, 1962.

7. Stone, O.J., and Mullins, F.J.: Role of Candida albicans in chronic disease. *Arch. Derm. 91*: 70-72, 1965.

8. Wittle, C.H., and Gersham, G.A.: Paronychia experimentally induced. *J. Invest. Derm. 40*: 267-269, 1963.

9. Ganor, S., and Pumpianski, R.: Chronic Candida albicans paronychia in adult Israeli women. *Brit. J. Derm. 90*: 77-83, 1974.

10. Stone, O.J., and Mullins, F.J.: Experimental studies on chronic paronychia. *Arch. Derm. 89*: 455-460, 1964.

11. Whittle, C.H., Moffatt, J.L., and Davis, R.A.: Paronychia or perionychia, aetiologic aspects. *Brit. J. Derm. 71*: 1-11, 1959.

12. Juhlin, L., and Liden, S.: Effect of Pimaricin in chronic paronychia. *Acta Derma-Venereol. 44*: 349-352, 1964.

13. Stone, O.J., and Mullins, F.J.: Incidence of chronic paronychia. *JAMA 186*: 71-73, 1963.

14. Stone, O.J., and Mullins, J.F.: Mechanisms of chronic paronychia in children. *Modern Med.* Oct. 21, 1968, p. 129.

15. Kerber, W.T., Reese, W.H., and Van Natla, J.: Balanitis, paronychia and onychia in a rhesus monkey. *Lab Animal Care 18*: 506-507, 1968.

16. Maibach, H.: Immediate hypersensitivity in hand eczema. Role of food-contact dermatitis. *Arch. Derm. 112*: 1289-1290, 1976.

17. **Krook, G.: Occupational dermatitis from Lactuca sativa (lettuce) and Cichorium (endive). Simultaneous occurances of immediate and delayed allergy as a course of contact dermatitis.** *Contact Dermatitis 3*: 27-36, 1977.

18. Sinha, S.M., Pasricha, J.S., Sharma, R.C., and Kandhari, K.C.: Vegetables responsible for contact dermatitis of the hands. *Arch. Derm. 113*: 776-779, 1977.

19. Mobacken, H., and Kregert, S.: Allergic contact dermatitis from cordomon. *Contact Dermatitis 1*: 175-176, 1975.

20. Hjorth, N.: Battery for testing of chefs and kitchen workers. *Contact Allergy 2*: 63, 1977.

CHAPTER 14

Psoriasis of the Nail

Nail involvement in psoriasis is common; reported incidences[1-5] vary from 10% to 50%. The clinical manifestations are multiple and varied, ranging from loosening of the nail plate to abnormal nail formation. Nail changes are more common on fingers than toes. Nail involvement as the sole manifestation of psoriasis is uncommon.

Psoriatic nail lesions in order of frequency are: pits, discoloration of nail bed, onycholysis, subungual keratosis, nail plate abnormalities, and splinter hemorrhages.

The histopathologic pattern seen in nail psoriasis is similar to that seen in skin psoriasis. Although the nail matrix and nail bed normally keratinize without a keratohyaline granular layer, the psoriatic changes seen in these structures can be well differentiated from the normal process.

PITS

Pits[6] are punctuate or irregular depressions (Figs. 1-3) which may form a pattern or be randomly spaced on the surface of the nail plate. They are the commonest lesion of nail psoriasis and vary in size, depth and shape. Shallow pits are not specific for psoriasis, being also associated with dermatitis, chronic eczematous dermatitis or alopecia areata. They are seen as well in individuals with no apparent disease. Deep pits, however, are characteristic for psoriasis.

Histopathology

Pits histologically represent defects in the superficial layers of the nail plate. The lining of the pit varies from normal nail plate cells to layers of parakeratotic cells. Pits situated distally (Fig. 6) on the nail plate contain few to no parakeratotic cells as compared to more proximally situated early pits (Figs. 4, 5, 7, 8) which usually contain mainly parakeratosis.

Fig. 9 diagrammatically shows that a psoriatic lesion in the proximal portion of the matrix gives rise to characteristic parakeratotic cells which are then carried outward as the result of nail plate growth. The actual pit results from desquamation of the poorly adherent abnormal parakeratotic focus as the nail plate moves distally beyond the proximal nail fold. The more distal the pit, the greater the chance of trauma to the surface of the nail, causing desquamation of the parakeratotic foci, and thus the fewer the parakeratotic cells that remain in the forming pit.

The proximal nail fold may also be responsible for pit formation, particularly that portion which is adjacent to the matrix. Fig. 10 is a diagrammatic drawing of the suggested mechanism of pit formation from the proximal nail fold (PNF).

DISCOLORATION–ONYCHOLYSIS

The location, shape and duration of the original psoriatic lesion in the nail bed or hyponychium will determine the resultant clinical appearance: e.g., a plaque which is entirely within the nail bed will result in an island of reddish discoloration under the nail plate (Fig. 11). A similar plaque in the hyponychium, medially or laterally, may result in a reddish spot and onycholysis (Fig. 12). Air under the separated nail plate imparts the whitish color exhibited by the nail plate over an onycholytic lesion (Fig. 13).

Histopathology

The histologic appearance of all these lesions is the same. Fig. 14 shows the psoriatic lesion in the nail bed seen in Fig. 11 characterized by thickening of the nail bed horny layer, marked parakeratosis, elongation of epidermal ridges and acanthosis of nail bed epidermis. There is a variable inflammatory response present in the lesion.

SUBUNGUAL KERATOSIS

Commonly seen in psoriasis as well as other nail diseases involving the hyponychium, subungual keratosis can have a variable clinical appearance. The accumulated subungual keratosis varies not only in amount but also in color. The uplifting of the nail plate depends on the extent and activity of the psoriatic process involving the hyponychium. The subungual keratosis may have a white-silvery color like the scales of skin psoriasis (Fig. 15) or, more commonly, a yellowish-greasy appearance (Fig. 16). The latter is not seen frequently in skin psoriasis. Often the subungual keratosis is dark brown or green. These cases are associated with a variety of microorganisms which are responsible for the discoloration.

Histopathology

The histology of the silvery-white type of subungual keratosis is similar to that seen in the nail bed lesions described previously (Fig. 14). The histology of the yellowish-greasy subungual keratotic lesions (Fig. 16) consists of the psoriatic process described previously, but there is an exaggerated inflammatory reaction (Figs. 17–20), with a large number of leukocytes, marked vasodilation, edema in the upper dermis, and a serum-like proteinaceous exudate. The exudate, which originates in the dermis (Fig. 20), appears to concentrate and fill cell spaces and forms large pools in the horny layer (Figs. 17, 18, 19). In hematoxylin- and eosin-stained sections, this material stains faintly and appears as pink hyaline amorphous masses of varying size between horny layer cells. The proteinaceous material is PAS-positive, diastase-resistant (Figs. 17, 18, 19) and produces a positive reaction with "the Danielli's" coupled tetrazonium reagent for the detection of aromatic amino acids (tyrosine, tryptophan, histidine) in tissues (Fig. 20). Histochemically, there is little evidence of acid mucopolysaccharides, fibrin, lipids, amyloid, or free aldehyde radicals prior to oxidation by periodic acid. This proteinaceous material most likely is serum or a serum glycoprotein. Often large amounts of the glycoprotein accumulate under the nail (Fig. 17). The described glycoprotein is a common occurrence in certain inflammatory diseases affecting the nail bed and hyponychium; among these are acute and chronic eczematous dermatitis, mycosis fungoides, acrodermatitis continua of Hallopeau, and Reiter's disease; in onychomycosis, however, it is strikingly absent.

Microbiologically, psoriasis poses an interesting dilemma. Why does one rarely find dermatophytes in a marked psoriatic subungual keratotic finger? Saprophytic air or soil-born contaminant fungi and yeasts, however, are common. Yeasts can be found with regularity in the accumulated subungual psoriatic horn. In toenails with psoriasis, however, one can occasionally culture a dermatophyte. This is an experience noted in Israel by Feuerman et al.,[7] rarely seen in Miami, Florida.

Bacterial colonization of the subungual debris with gram-positive micrococci and Pseudomonas aeruginosa is also common.

SEVERE NAIL PLATE ABNORMALITIES

In severe psoriatic nail involvement, it is not uncommon to have a whitish, crumbly, deformed nail plate marked by numerous transverse grooves and furrows (Figs. 21, 22, 25–27).

Histopathology

The histologic process is seen in Fig. 23; matrix and proximal nail fold are involved with psoriasis and exhibit the characteristic parakeratosis, acanthosis, etc. The nail plate produced consists of parakeratotic cells, crumbling easily. This can be seen clinically in Fig. 25; a marker near the large scaling of the nail plate (NP) can be followed to show the latter as a large transverse furrow.

SPLINTER HEMORRHAGES

These commonly seen in psoriasis (Fig. 24). They have been described in detail[8] and characteristically are seen only in the nail bed (see Ch. XVIII).

TREATMENT OF PSORIATIC NAILS

Today, there is no easy, effective method to treat nail psoriasis. There are topicals, radiation, injections, and systemic medications, but all have problems. The patient must be highly motivated. The treatment must have a great advantage over the treatment time invested by the patient since the disease may recur shortly after treatment is stopped.

Topicals

There is no topical medication presently used which can penetrate the nail plate and effectively deliver a therapeutic dose to the underlying matrix or nail bed. Topical corticosteroids, 5-flurouracil, and retinoic acid are variably effective because they do not treat the site involved. Naturally, the proximal nail fold and hyponychium are the most easily treated. Nail plate avulsion can accomplish good treatment response, but is it worth it when the disease may recur one week after the nail plate grows out? In my hands, topical treatment is so variable that it is minimally effective. The use of topically applied antimetabolites such as 5-flurouracil, methotrexate and merchlorethanime[9] seems to be effective but incurs morbidity problems and therefore is impractical.

Intralesional Corticosteroids

Either by Dermojet[10] or injected intralesionally[11], corticosteroids work miracles. Lesions clear—only to recur. Patients are willing at first, then desist after painful injections continue for periods of months thereafter. The dose should not exceed 2.5 mg/cc.

Antimetabolites

Excellent results can be obtained by Methotrexate (Fig. 30) or mycophenolic acid (Figs. 28, 29) as well as any other drug in that category. Usually, widespread disease and severe arthritis are prerequisites.

PUVA compares to antimetabolite treatment. The nails now become very melanotic (see Ch. XIX, Fig. 6).

Recently, Hoffman et al.[13] have developed a high intensity light device which could be used for PUVA of psoriatic nails.

PUSTULAR PSORIASIS OF THE NAIL UNIT

This entity may present as the sole psoriatic manifestation more commonly than it concurs with psoriasis elsewhere. I have seen a child with one nail involved (biopsy proven) (Fig. 31), an adult female with one lesion recurrent (Fig. 32), another adult female with various fingernails and toenails involved (Figs. 33–35), and a young female with all ten fingernails so severely pustular that the entire nail plates were lifted out of their beds (Fig. 36). None of these patients had skin psoriasis elsewhere. Cutting the uplifted nail plate (Fig. 37) revealed widespread explosive pustular psoriasis. Fig. 38 shows a patient with widespread psoriasis and pustular nail unit psoriasis.

Treatment of Pustular Psoriasis

The treatment of pustular psoriasis is very discouraging. I have compared 5-flurourocil vs. retinoic acid vs. injectable steroids, and all lesions behave the same way—they come and go according to their own dispositions.

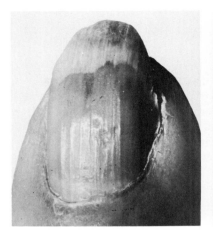

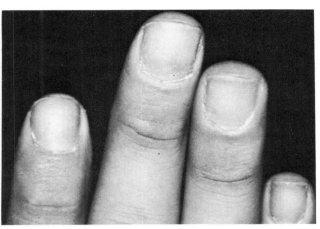

Fig. 1. Pits on surface of nail plate. (University of Miami) (Zaias, *Arch. Derm.* 99: 571, 1969, Fig. 7)

Fig. 2. Psoriasis of nails only. Very small pits throughout surface of nails.

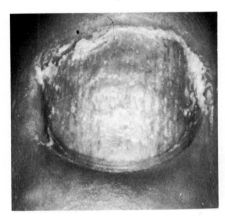

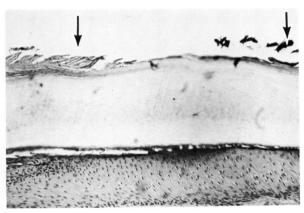

Fig. 3. Psoriasis of nails only. Close-up of patient in Fig. 2. Nails of other hand showed similar pits on the surface.

Fig. 4. Photomicrograph, longitudinal section of pits on surface of nail plate (arrows). H&E X120.

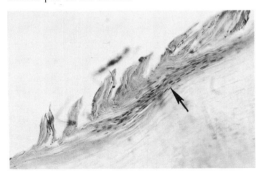

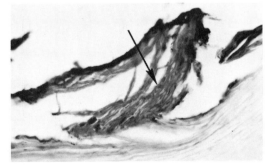

Fig. 5. Photomicrograph, longitudinal section of pit. Focus of parakeratosis (arrow up) in nail plate which will become a pit when it falls off. Note that the cuticle (stratum corneum of proximal nail fold) sandwiches the focus of abnormal cells with the nail plate. H&E X120. (Zaias, *Arch. Derm.* 99: 572, 1969. Fig. 10)

Fig. 6. More distal focus of cells has fallen out. Slight remnants of this focus are seen (arrow). H&E X240. (Zaias, *Arch. Derm.* 99: 571, 1969, Fig. 8)

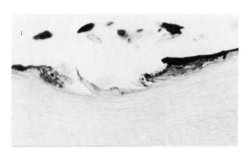

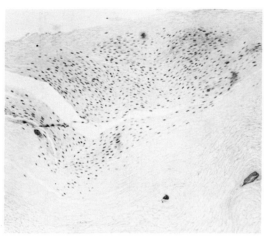

Fig. 7. Paraketatotic foci of cells now being shed. Formation of pit. H&E X120. (Zaias, *Arch. Derm. 99*: 571, 1969, Fig. 9)

Fig. 8. Parakeratotic focus is a little deeper in nail plate than previous pits. This will form deeper pit. H&E X120. Zaias, *Arch. Derm. 99*: 572, Fig. 9)

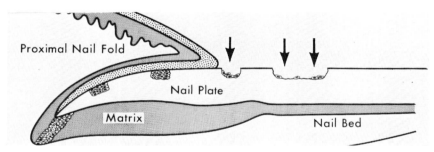

Fig. 9. Diagrammatic drawing summarizing formation of pit due to minuscule papule of psoriasis measuring as little as a millimeter in proximal matrix and moving distally (arrow down). Length of pit is function of duration of papule in matrix. Lesion (double arrow) existed 2–3 times as long as first pit (arrow). (Zaias, *Arch. Derm. 99*: 573, 1969, Fig. 13)

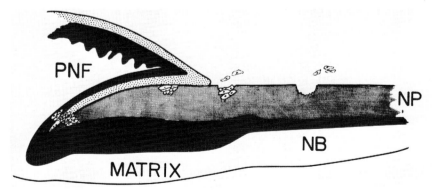

Fig. 10. Diagrammatic drawing of possible mechanism of pit formation through lesion in proximal area of proximal nail fold due to psoriasis or any eczematosis dermatitis. (Zaias, *Arch. Derm. 99*: 574, 1969, Fig. 16)

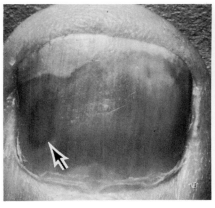

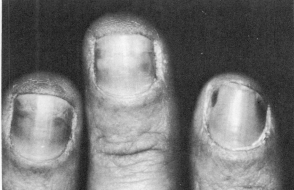

Fig. 11. Nail bed psoriatic papule, reddish yellow in appearance; when it involves hyponychial area, onycholysis can be seen clinically.

Fig. 12. Psoriatic onycholysis.

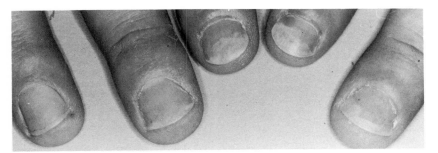

Figure 13. Psoriatic onycholysis (nail bed and hyponychial psoriasis). Often Candida albicans may colonize subungual niche.

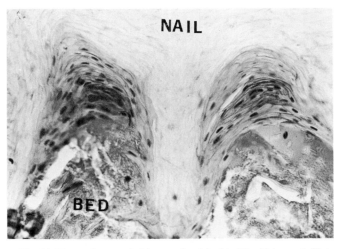

Fig. 14. Photomicrograph, biopsy of nail bed in Fig. 11 (arrow). Note psoriatic confluent parakeratosis. H&E X480.

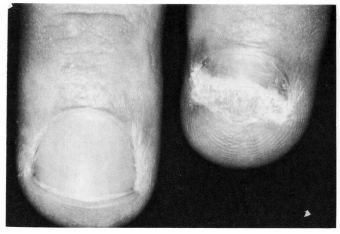

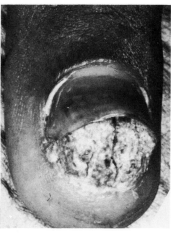

Fig. 15. Psoriasis of one nail only. Subungual keratosis is dry, its scale silvery in color.

Fig. 16. Psoriasis of one nail, adolescent female, nail bed and hyponychium involved. Characteristic serum-laden reddish hyperkeratotis lesion.

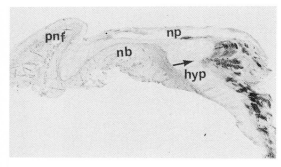

Fig. 17. Photomicrograph, biopsy of psoriatic nail (nail bed and hyponychium) showing possible explanation for yellowish-red color of lesion (arrow). P.A.S. X26. Note dark material, higher magnification in Fig. 18. (Zaias *Arch. Derm. 99*: 575, 1969, Fig. 21)

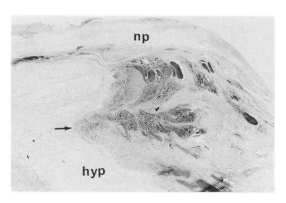

Fig. 18. Higher magnification of Fig. 17. Arrow shows serum-like material among keratinocytes of hyponychium. P.A.S. X180: (Zaias, *Arch. Derm. 99*: 575, 1969, Fig. 22)

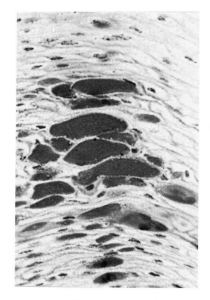

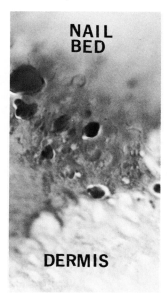

Fig. 20. Serum-like material seems to originate from dermis and is deposited among keratinocytes of nail bed epidermis. P.A.S. X800. (Zaias, *Arch. Derm. 97*: 576, 1969. Fig. 24)

Fig. 19. Higher magnification of Fig. 18. P.A.S. X600.

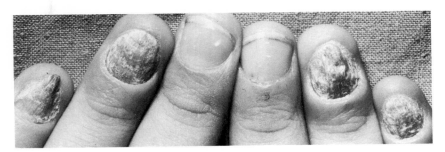

Fig. 21. Psoriasis of proximal matrix mostly. Note sharing of two fingers. Damage to nail plate is only superficial.

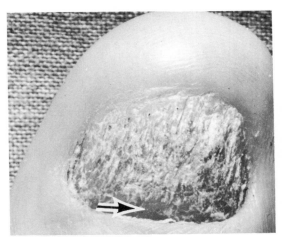

Fig. 22. Psoriasis mainly of proximal matrix. Patient is now in remission. Note new nail plate (arrows).

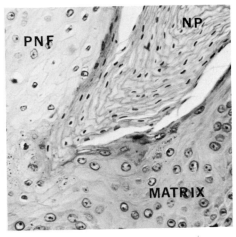

Fig. 23. Photomicrograph, biopsy showing psoriatic involvement of proximal areas of PNF and matrix. Nail plate is made up of parakeratotic onychocytes. H&E X480. (Zaias, *Arch. Derm. 99:* 578, 1969, Fig. 31)

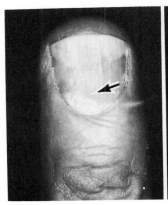

Fig. 24. Proximal matrix; psoriasis nail lesions (arrow).

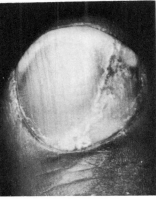

Fig. 25. Proximal matrix; psoriasis nail lesion, three months (Zaias, *Arch. Derm. 99:* 577, 1969, Fig. 30)

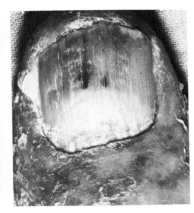

Fig. 26. Psoriasis: subungual hemorrhages. (Zaias, *Arch. Derm. 99:* 577, 1969, Fig. 30)

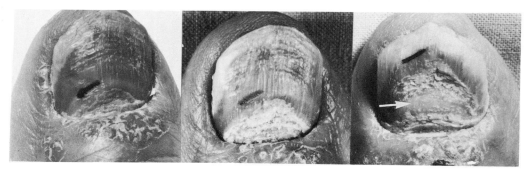

Fig. 27. a. Course of psoriatic plaque of proximal matrix can be seen in appearance of nail plate. Below the **mark, early appearance of nail plate lesion. b. Two weeks later, plaque is still active. c. Two months later, sur**face of nail plate reflects periodicity of active-remissive psoriasis of proximal matrix; arrow shows normal nail plate—no psoriasis. Every 2–3 weeks this patient had an active lesion. (Zaias, *Arch. Derm. 99:* 577, 1969. Fig. 30)

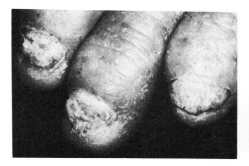

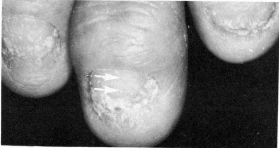

Fig. 28. Psoriatic arthritis with onychopsoriasis.

Fig. 29. Normal nail plate after mycophenolic acid treatment three months (arrow).

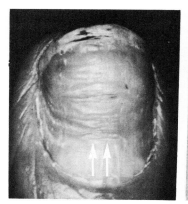

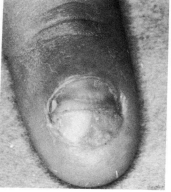

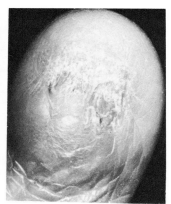

Fig. 30. Normal nail growth following Methotrexate. Of all antimetabolites treatments, I believe Methotrexate is most satisfactory for nails and joints.

Fig. 31. Pustular psoriasis, one nail only, in child.

Fig. 32. Pustular psoriasis, one nail only, in 60-year-old female. Nail plate shed.

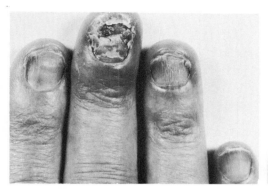

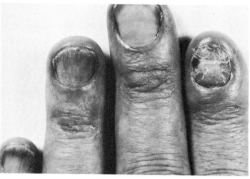

Fig. 33. Pustular psoriasis in patient with only two fingernails involved and one toenail.

Fig. 34. Patient in Fig. 33.

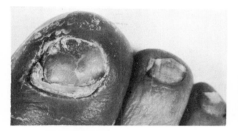

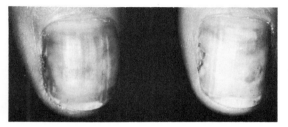

Fig. 35. Patient in Figure 33; great toe, right.

Fig. 36. Pustular psoriasis of nail bed, massive and confluent, producing lysis of all ten fingernails only, in 25-year-old female.

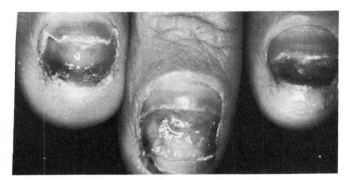

Fig. 37. Nail plates cut off patient in Fig. 36 to show extent of involvement.

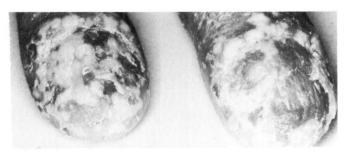

Fig. 38. Pusutlar psoriasis of skin and nails. Nail plate shed.

NOTES

1. Heller, J.: *Die Krankheiten der Nagel.* Berlin: Hirschwald, 1900.

2. Crawford, G.M.: Psoriasis of the nails. *Arch. Derm. Syph. 38*: 583-594, 1938.

3. Pardo-Castello, V., and Pardo, O.A.: *Diseases of the Nails.* Springfield, Ill: Charles C. Thomas, 1960.

4. Calvert, H.T., Smith, M.A., and Wells, R.S.: Psoriasis and the nails. *Brit. J. Derm. 76*: 415-418, 1963.

5. Baker, H., Golding, D.N., and Thompson, M.: The nails in psoriatic arthritis. *Brit. J. Derm. 76*: 549-554, 1964.

6. Alkiewicz, J.: Psoriasis of the nail. *Brit. J. Derm. 60*: 195-200, 1948.

7. Feuerman, E., Alteras, I., and Aryelly, J.: The incidence of pathogenic fungi in psoriatic nails. *Castellania 4*: 195-196, 1976.

8. Kuske, H.: Splitterblutungen der Nagel Platte, *Dermatologica 123*: 219-226, 1961.

9. Notowicz, A., Stolz, E., and Heuvel, N.V.D.: Treatment of Hallopeau's acrodermatitis with topical mechlorethamine. *Arch. Derm. 114*: 129, 1978.

10. Litt, J.Z.: Severe nail dystrophy: treatment with Dermo-Jet injections of triancinolone acetonide. *Cutis 8*: 569-571, 1971.

11. Peachey, R.D.G., Pye, R.J., and Harman, R.R.M.: Treatment of psoriatic nail dystrophy with intra dermal steroid injections. *Brit. J. Derm. 95*: 75-78, 1977.

12. Zaias, N.: Psoriasis of the nail. *Arch. Derm. 99*: 567-579, 1966.

13. Hofman, C., Plewig, G., and Braun-falco, O.: Photochemotherepy nail psoriasis. *Int. Psoriasis Bull. 4*: 3-4, 1977.

CHAPTER 15

Onycholysis

Onycholysis is defined as the separation of the nail plate from the nail bed. When this occurs, air entering from the distal free edge gives the separated nail plate the visual image of opaque white (Figs. 1, 3, 6). Onycholysis occurs very frequently in fingernails, less so in toenails. This is a women's disease seen only in males who have distinctive jobs relating to the water-borne environment, e.g., janitors, bartenders, fruit juice squeezers, tropical fish farmers, strawberry farmers and pickers; barbers also suffer with onycholysis as an occupational hazard.

The remarks that follow are made in reference to women's onycholysis. There are no exact statistics on the incidence of onycholysis, but one of every ten patients seen at my office is seen for this disease. These are females varying from age twenty-five on, peaking at the fifty-to-sixty age group.

Clinically, a green color (Fig. 5) accompanies the onycholysis in about 50% of cases. This is due to pyocyanin, a water-insoluble pigment of Pseudomonas aeruginosa. More will be said about this later.

The most commonly recognized pathogen is Candida albicans, which can be isolated in 74% of the cases (see Table I). For a moment, let us theorize that C. albicans is a primary causal agent in onycholysis. How it produces the separation is not clear, but it is known that the yeast (C. albicans) can occur in the gastrointestinal tract of roughly 40–50% of people over twenty years old. Furthermore, in women, it is conceivable and very probable that the gastrointestinal tract seeds the vagina.[1] The mouth may also serve as a reservoir site. Some women have a symptomatic vaginitis, but in others the organism may be isolated in spite of the absence of symptoms (see Table II). The fingers then are probably seeded by both gastrointestinal and vaginal sites. Thus treatment of all three sites at the same time may be curative for patients who suffer recurrent onycholysis or vaginitis.

DIAGNOSIS AND TREATMENT

The most important treatment "act" is to cut off all the onycholytic nail (Figs. 1, 2). This will:

1. Permit taking material from the most proximal lytic area for diagnosis (smear stained by Gram's method).

2. Expose the nail bed to air and dry it, which is crucial in the fight against C. albicans and other bacteria which inhabit the "Lytic Hotel," i.e., Pseudomonas (Figs. 6–9).

3. Enable the clinician to apply the treatment to the most proximal areas of the nail bed, where the disease is most active.

All antibiotics that are anticandidal can be used: nystatin, clotrimazole, miconazole, haloprogin. Every month, the patient returns for further cutting of whatever nail plate grew unattached (usually 1–2 mm). By the second month, very little, if any, nail plate grows unattached. The patient then continues to apply the antibiotic until all the nails look normal (Fig. 4).

Nails containing Pseudomonas (green) need not be treated with anti-Pseudomonas medication as the nail cutting (dry environment) will suffice. It is important that the patient not wear band-aids, gloves or such occlusive devices. Cleaning the nail with a soft brush, using soap and water is encouraged. Green nails sometimes do not grow Pseudomonas; this usually signifies that the bacterium has died off and left the pyocyanin-stained nail in days of life. This fact has led to erroneous descriptions of green yeast and green aspergillus nail infections. Other yeasts have been isolated from onycholytic nails; proof of pathogenicity is still needed (see Table I). Non-microbial onycholysis has been described these are summarized in Table III.

Table 1
Yeast Isolated from 100 Onycholytic Nails

	Negroni (1971)	Zapater & Rudich (1969) (% of cases)	Zaias
Candida tropicalis	33	28	
Candida parapsilosis	30	14	
Canadida albicans	28	52	74
Trichosporon cutaneum	3		
Candida solani	3		

Table II
Correlation of Recovery of Candida albicans and Pseudomonas Aeruginosa from Nails and Vagina in 106 Patients

C. albicans culture positive from nails with *asymptomatic culture negative vagina*	44 (41.5%)	Nurse, nail dystrophy, stewardness, lacquer dermatitis, compulsiver cleaner, finger sucker, psoriasis, liver cirrhosis
C. albicans culture positive from nails with *asymptomatic culture positive vagina*	28 (26.4%)	Oral surgeons nurse, diabetes
C. albicans culture positive from nails with *symptomatic culture positive* C. albicans vaginitis	6 (5.7%)	
Nail culture *negative* Vaginal culture *negative*	*28* (26.4%) ——————— 106	6 grew out Pseudomonas aeruginosa

Table III
Nonmicrobiological Onycholysis

Thyroid disease
Bantu porphyria
Erythropoetic protoporphyria
Photosensitivity (phototoxic to drugs)
Pellagra
Porphyria cutanea tarda

(See discussion of onycholysis in Ch. 22)

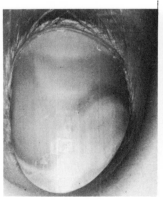 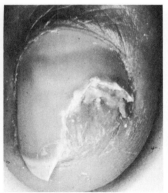 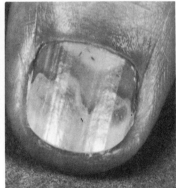

Fig. 1. Onycholysis by Candida albicans in 20-year-old female patient.

Fig. 2. Nail plate cut away to show subungual material from which specimen will be taken for culture and gram stain. Recommended amount of nail plate to be cut in treatment, so whatever cream patient receives will not reach most remote recess of "lytic" space.

Fig. 3. Onycholysis by Candida albicans, 25-year-old female.

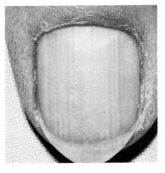

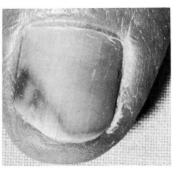

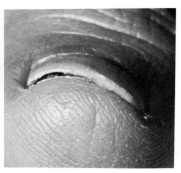

Fig. 4. Same patient cured 4 months later. Nail plate cut as in Fig. 2, every 3–4 weeks, and anti-Candida medicaton applied b.i.d. Gloves should be discouraged.

Fig. 5. Onycholysis, 55-year-old female. Candida albicans and Pseudomonas aeruginosa.

Fig. 6. Note thinning of nail-plate typical for Pseudomonas.

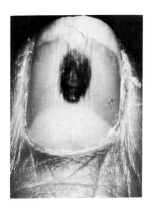

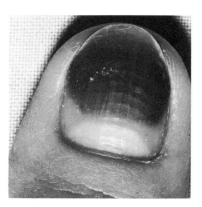

Fig. 7. Pseudomonas onycholysis. Usually, Pseudomonas colonizes an already available space; once under nail plate, however, it spreads rapidly. Colors may vary from chartreuse to near-black.

Fig. 8. Extensive Pseudomonas onycholysis. It is doubtful that Pseudomonas is a primary pathogen in onycholysis. Often it will stain the nail plate, Pyocyonin, and at some time thereafter the Pseudomonas will die off, leaving a green nail with negative culture.

NOTES

1. Miles, M., Olsen, L., and Rogers, A.: Recurrent vaginal candidiasis. *JAMA 238*: 1836-1837, 1977.
2. Zapater, R.C., and Rudich, R.N.: Onicomicosis de mano. *Arch. Argent. Dermat. 29*: 183-187, 1969.
3. Negroni, R.: Yeasts isolated from onycholytic nails. *Dermatologia 13*: 353-363, 1971.

CHAPTER 16

Bacterial Diseases
Affecting the Nail Unit

PSEUDOMONAS

Bacteria, generally, are not gifted biochemically to attack the nail plate. A notable exception is Pseudomonas aeruginosa, a gram-negative bacterium with the greatest capability to break down nail plate. I have already discussed how onycholysis populated by Pseudomonas results in a widening and thinning of the nail plate. Naturally, conditions must be propitious for the bacteria to multiply. The clinical picture's, not of onycholysis or paronychia, but rather of involvement of the superior and ventral surface of the nail plate (Figs. 1, 2, 3). In Fig. 1, the entire surface was colonized by Pseudomonas, which left its characteristic calling card, pyocyanin.[1] The patient, a diabetic who did normal housework, had had this problem for 6 months. Fig. 2 is a diabetic patient with osteoarthritis. The figure shows greenish areas originating in the lateral nail fold. This condition is very difficult to treat. Fig. 3 shows another patient with multiple foci of pseudomonas.

How does the bacterium get under the small areas of the lateral and proximal nail folds? Why does it not produce a reaction in the proximal nail fold? Is it really a causative agent? All these are unanswered question.

Treatment

The treatment—before a patient showed me how to cure this disease—was to avulse the nail plate. Today, I follow Mrs. K's advice: Clorox, diluted one-to-four, a few drops applied three times a day. The results are shown in Fig. 1 (arrow), which is Mrs. K's nail.

DIPHTHEROIDS AND CORYNEBACTERIA

The bacteria which, so far, have not produced a clinically recognized disease of the nail are the diphtheroids and, in particular, the corynebacteria. Members of this genus are responsible for diseases in which the target site is the horny layer of the skin and hair, i.e.:

Trichomycosis axillaris	Hair	C. tenuis
Erythrasma	Stratum corneum	C. minutissimun
Pitted keratolysis	Palmar-plantar Stratum corneum	C. corynebacteria

Corynebacterium minutessimun has recently been described to be associated with the clinical picture of distal subungual onychomycosis.[2] No dermatophyte was isolated from the diseased nail but a bacterium which was was characterized as C. minutissimun was isolated from the subungal debris in 17 cases.

The possibility exists for a diphtheroid or corynebacterium to produce a D.S.O.-like picture. Table I shows data from a study[3] of subungual distal abnormalities in 183 toenails. The surprising facts were that dermatophytes were recovered in only 23% of the abnormal nails and no fungi of any kind were recovered in 27% of those nails. The predominant bacteria (aerobic) were the diphtheroids. Thus it is possible that they play a role as nail pathogens. This, however, needs further proof.

Table 1

Recovery of Dermatophytes Molds, Yeasts and Bacteria from 183 Subungual Keratotic Toenails (not Psoriatic)

			Direct Microscopic Examinations (KOH)
			Total % Positive
Organism Isolated	%Positive	% Negative	and Negative
Dermatophytes	18.1	4.1	22.7
Molds and yeasts	16.2	33.1	49.3
Bacteria only	6.7	21.3	28
Total	41.0	59.0	100.0

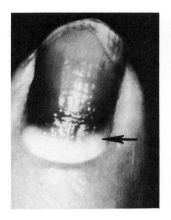

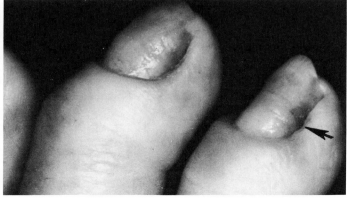

Fig. 1. Pseudomonas over surface of nail. Proximally located white area is new noninvolved nail plate. Treatment: Clorox diluted 1:10 produced cure.

Fig. 2. Pseudomonas over surface in nail pf patient with diabetes. Arthritic changes resulted in deformed nail plate. Not infrequently complex; very hard to cure.

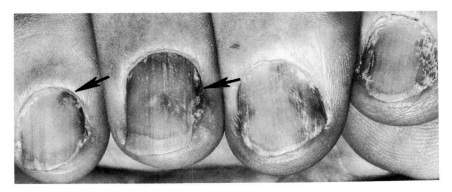

Fig. 3. Psoriasis and Pseudomonas over surface of nail plate.

NOTES

1. Shellow, W.V.R., and Koplon, B.S.: Green striped nails: chromonychia due to Pseudomonas aeruginosa. *Arch. Derm. 97*: 149-153, 1968.
2. Negroni, P.: Erythrasma of the nails. *Med. Cut., I.L.A. No. 5*: 349-358, 1976.
3. Zaias, N.: Onychomycosis. *Arch. Derm. 105*: 263-274, 1972.

CHAPTER 17

Nail Unit Dystrophy
Not Related to Any Systemic Disorder

PINCER, TRUMPET OR OMEGA NAILS

This nail plate dystrophy is commonly seen in toenails. The nail plate arises from under the proximal nail fold normally, but shortly afterward (distally) it becomes laterally compressed. The nail plate lateral compression may vary from minimal amounts (Figs. 1, 2) or result in the formation of a cylinder (Fig. 3, 4); hence the various terms pincer, trumpet or omega given to this dystrophy.

Although the etiology of this condition is unknown in toenails, it is suspected to be secondary to the wearing of shoes. In fingernails, it is associated with osteoarthritic changes of the distal interphalangeal joint. Possibly the fibrous deposits around this joint replace the lateral areas of the matrix medially, producing a laterally compressed nail plate. A shoe-related dystrophy and a matrix architectural displacement can be differentiated by looking at the newly emerging nail plate. In the latter, the nail plate emerges normally flat (Fig. 3); in the former, the compression of the lateral nail plate is already visible at its emergence from under the proximal nail fold (Fig. 2).

Treatment for matrix displacement is very unsatisfactory; however, in cases suspected to be caused by footwear, avulsion of the nail plate will allow an architectural realignment of the entrapped nail bed between the lateral aspects of the nail plate. At times, a first avulsion succeeds only in a moderate correction, requiring a second avulsion for a completely normal nail plate. Avulsion should not require surgical excisions at lateral borders of proximal nail folds, but rather blunt avulsion (see Ch. 6). Usually, this dystrophy is asymptomatic.

ONYCHOMANIA

A series of nail plate abnormalities will be described which are self-perpetuating and may also be self-induced. The typical patient is intense, highly motivated, and so meticulous and compulsive that he may produce the lesion while treating and caring for his nail's health.

Median Nail Plate Dystrophy

Under the term dystrophia mediana canaliformis are a series of different deformities all having in common damage at some point in the proximal matrix, so that, over a period of time, a longitudinal defect is noted on the nail plate (NP) (Figs. 5–10). It does not have to be mid-line (Fig. 6). The width of the defect is determined by the width of the matrix damage (Fig. 10). The deformity is usually self-made due to tic or habit, and often the patient does not realize that he himself is causing the deformity of the nail. These dystrophies are temporary, improving and worsening (arrow, Fig. 5).

Sculptured Onycholysis

This is another manifestation of a self-perpetuating nail abnormality. The clue lies in the shape of the proximal border of the lysis; normally, the proximal lytic border is not linear, scalloped or geometric but gently curved (Figs. 11–13). The other clue is the dead white opaque color of the lytic portion of the nail (Fig. 13). This is produced by scraping, etc., the underside of the nail plate with a sharp instrument.

Swirl Nail Plate Deformity

This deformity is self-created by the patient's running one fingertip pad across the nail plate of another finger (Fig. 16).

Artefactual Appearance of Nail Defects

The patient presents defects which are not physiologically feasible. Fig. 14 shows a linear tear (arrow) in the middle fingernail; note the lesion beginning on the same finger of the other hand. Fig. 15 shows a defect of the surface of the nail plate (NP)—a partial interrupted swirl.

Permanent Nail Unit Damage for Special Purposes

Destruction of the nail unit due to the nail plate's interference with making a tight fist is shown in Figs. 17–19. This was an excision of the matrix area of all fingers. The patient wanted to obtain the title of Iron Palm or Black Glove—a karate discipline in which the subject strikes his clenched fist into a cylinder filled with sand. A certain depth must be achieved for the title. The arrow in Fig. 19 indicates a neuroma. The arrow up in Fig. 18 shows a callus made by constant clenching of the fist.

Severe Nail Biting

Nail biting, generally very commonplace, is usually a "nervous" habit which produces minimal damage to the distal edge of the nail plate. In severe nail biting, damage to the proximal nail fold (PNF) and the matrix results in a ptergium (arrow, Fig. 20).

Schizophrenic Behavior

The patient in Figs. 21 and 22 is a paranoid schizophrenic who bit her nails to the bone. This is also seen in demented children with Lisch-Nyhan or similar disorders, who eat everything they can put in their mouth.

Accidental Dystrophy

The custom, originating from superstition, of not cutting a baby's fingernails and/or placing mittens on the baby to prevent him from scratching has been reported to result in gangrene and loss of the affected portion of the digit.[1] Loose threads in the mitten may become tightly entwined around the infant's finger, remaining unnoticed until the constriction has done severe damage.

ONYCHOGRYPHOSIS

This dystrophy is most likely caused by the shoe or footgear (classically, the pointed-toe shoe) since the bend of all nails is toward the median of the foot (arrows, Fig. 23; Figs. 24, 26, 27). The nail plate grows hypertrophied (Fig. 21) and unevenly at the matrix. One side of the matrix grows faster than the other (Fig. 26); the faster growing side will determine the direction of the deformity. Looking clinically like a ram's horn, the nail bed is also hypertrophied. Treatment is the complete destruction of the matrix—preferably by phenol.

Onychoschizia

This layering of the nail plate is not an uncommon abnormality (Fig. 28). Absolutely nothing is known about it.

Ridging

It is not unusual to see longitudinal ridges in the nail plate after the age of twenty-nine (arrows, Fig. 29). These are asymptomatic and are a bother to the patient only as a curiosity or as a cosmetic concern. The cause is unknown.

Brittle Nails

This subject has, indeed, created a great interest among the lay population as well as among scientists. Usually noted in forty- to sixty-year-old women, it can be divided into two categories: (1) a history of always having had brittle nails and (2) a sudden onset in adulthood or post-menopause. If the patient has always had brittle nails, she will continue to have them. In contrast, patients who recently acquired brittle nails will have normal nails again; the brittle nails may last as long as four years but will normalize by themselves. There is no available treatment that is proven effective.[2]

Ectopic Nail

This usually follows trauma to the nail matrix. A small portion of matrix produces a nail outside the proximal nail fold (Fig. 31).

Koilonychia (Spoon Nails) (Acquired)

The normal contour of the nail plate is slightly convex from one lateral nail fold to the other. In koilonychia, this normal contour is not only lost but becomes a concavity (Fig. 30). The condition may be associated with anemia. See Pulmer Vinson's syndrome, Ch. 22, and Polycythemia.[3]

Dystrophyic Fifth Toenail

It is extremely common among the population to have the fifth toenail dystrophic— usually gnarled and unrecognizable as a nail plate, like a spicule of horn. Histopathologically, the nail unit has stretched out and the proximal nail fold is scanty. The matrix has lost its diagonally distal keratinization direction, and its direction now is perpendicular with the surface of the digit. Fig. 32 shows such a toe. Note the minimal PNF (short arrow); the matrix is recognizable only by having unstained "nail plate" horn originating from it (area between arrows). The nail bed is also active, producing large quantities of horn (large arrow).

Nail Damage Caused by Weed Killers and Insecticides

Samman[11] was first aware of the unusual changes that paraquat and diquat produced to the nail. These changes consisted in a nail which looked like a half-and-half nail (Fig. 36).

Lichen Striatus

Lichen Striatus with nail involvement was described by Kaufman as the fourth reported case in the literature[24] (Figs. 33, 34).

Epidermal Nevus[5]

This lesion histologically proven from proximal nail fold skin must have affected the proximal matrix and caused the nail plate deformity in Fig. 35.

Twenty Nail Dystrophy of Childhood[6]

Twenty nail plates all with superficial striations, which occurs in children eighteen months to eighteen years is indeed interesting. It is self-healing as the child matures and is not accompanied by any other signs of dermatologic disease. Clinically its indistinguishible from lichen planus

Biopsies of minimally involved twenty nail dystrophy cases histologically are lichen planus; I therefore recommend that the term "twenty nail dystrophy of children" be dropped and the disease recognized as another sign of lichen planus.

Baran[7] published this sign associated with alopecia areata and had one patient with a hereditary syndrome featuring abnormal hair growth whose nails also looked identical. See Chapter 12.

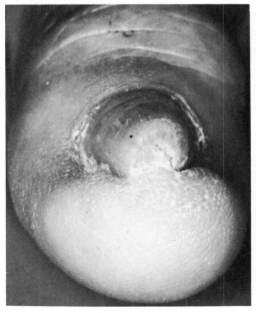

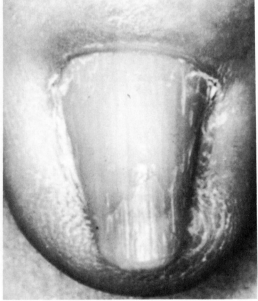

Fig. 1. Pincer nail of finger. Patient has osteoarthritis, which probably makes matrix's dropped position over the phalanx more convex. Note nail plate emerging strongly laterally compressed.

Fig. 2. Top view of nail in Fig. 1.

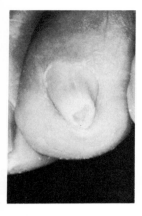

Fig. 3. Pincer toenail. Despite marked abnormality, toes are usually asymptomatic.

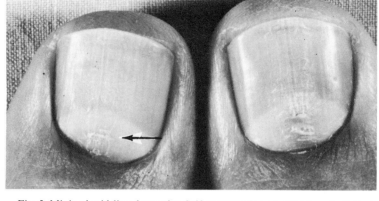

Fig. 5. Minimal mid-line dystrophy. Self-perpetuating on right thumb. Patient just began to work his left thumb (arrow).

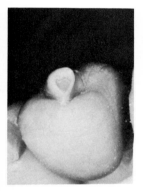

Fig. 4. Note flattened normal emerging nail plate. Compresses laterally from pressure of shoe-clad environment. Avulsion helpful.

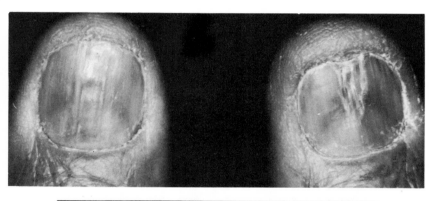

Fig. 7. & 8. Median dystrophy. Remarkable nail plate abnormality. Self-perpetuating.

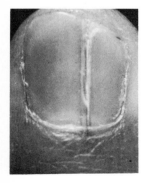

Fig. 6. Para-median dystrophy. Defect appears to be on matrix, yet avulsion resulted in new, normal nail plate.

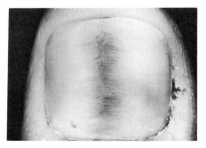

Fig. 9. Self-perpetuating. Pushing of PNF of thumb and index finger.

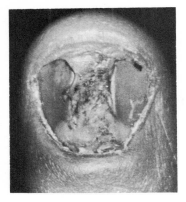

Fig. 10. Same as Fig. 5, but more severe.

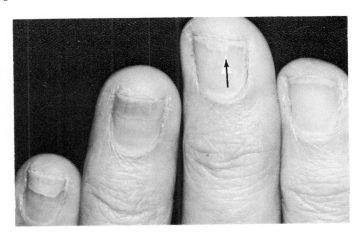

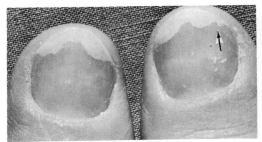

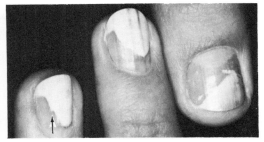

Fig. 11, 12 and 13. Artifactual (sculptured) onychoysis. Arrow shows unnatural separation.

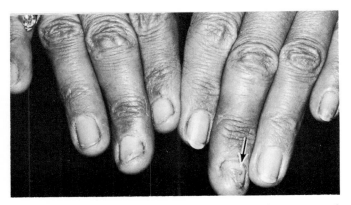

Fig. 14. Self-perpetuating nail abnormality. Arrow shows unnatural
shape of defect. Note middle fingernails of both hands involved.

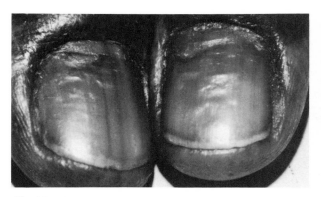

Fig. 15. Minimal changes; self-made.

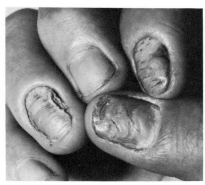

Fig. 16. Swirl grooving, caused by pressure on both lateral edges of nail plate. PNF also has to be stroked.

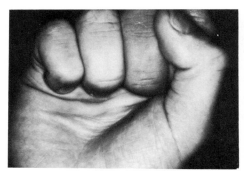

Fig. 17. Clenched fist of patient in karate pose.

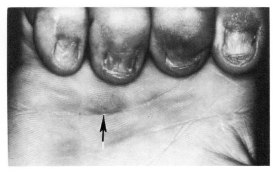

Fig. 18. Nail beds devoid of nail matrix and plates due to surgical removal of matrices. Arrow up, callouses produced by pushing fingertip into palm.

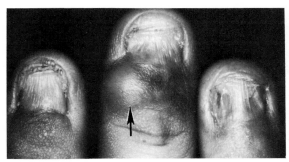

Fig. 19. Neuroma secondary to matrix excision and subsequent trauma.

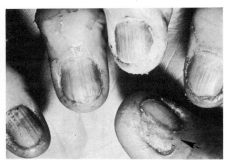

Fig. 20. Neurotic patient. Self-destructive.

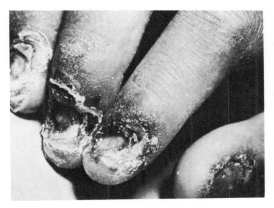

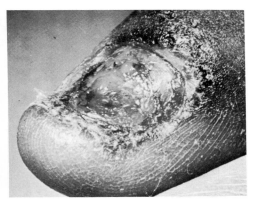

Fig. 21. Psychotic patient. Self-destructive.

Fig. 22. Another finger of patient in Fig. 21.

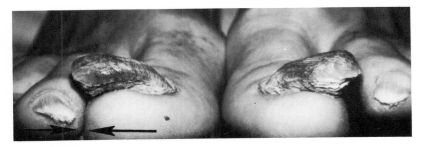

Fig. 23. Onychogryphosis. Note direction of nail plate. Probably result of pressure of shoe-clad environment.

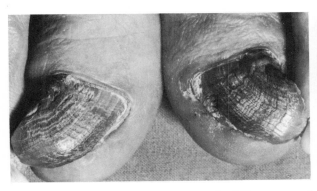

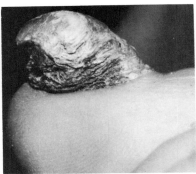

Fig. 24. Onychogryphosis. (University of Miami, Department of Dermatology)

Fig. 25. Onychogryphosis with nail bed hyperplasia.

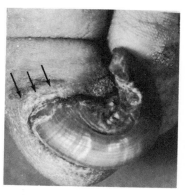

Fig. 26. Severe onychogryphosis. Note that one side of matrix (arrow) is producing normal nail plate while other side is not producing nail plate, thus making nail grow in that direction.

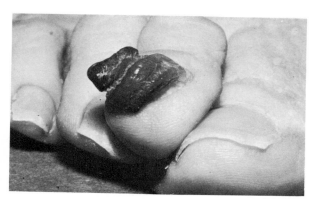

Fig. 27. Ram's horn onychogryphosis.

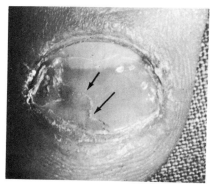

Fig. 28. Onychoschizia. Distal layering of nail plate. (University of Miami, Department of Dermatology)

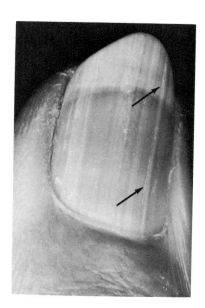

Fig. 29. Longitudinal ridge usually seen without underlying disease in older patients.

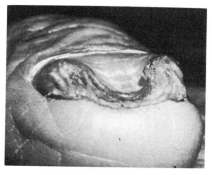

Fig. 30. Koilonychia secondary to onychomycosis. (University of Miami, Department of Dermatology)

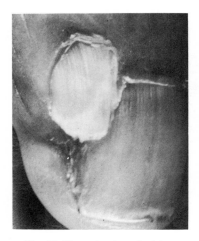

Fig. 31. Heterotropic nail plate secondary to trauma. (Courtesy Dr. Orville Stone)

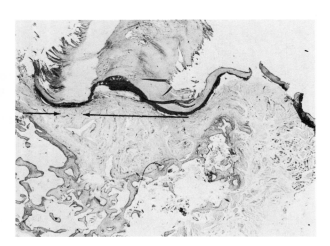

Fig. 32. Photomicrograph, dystrophic fifth toenail showing flattened proximal nail fold (PNF) (small arrow). Nail bed is producing horny layer (long arrow). Nail matrix (space between arrow heads) produces transparent nail plate. H&E X42.

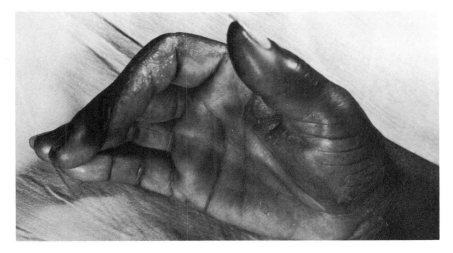

Fig. 33. Lichen striatus in 10-year-old female, involving finger.

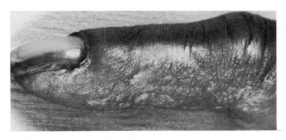

Fig. 34. Patient in Fig. 33, showing nail matrix involvement with nail plate dystrophy and hyperpigmentations. Noted in two patients.

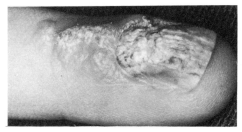

Fig. 35. Epidermal nevus, biophs proven, nail plate dystrophy.

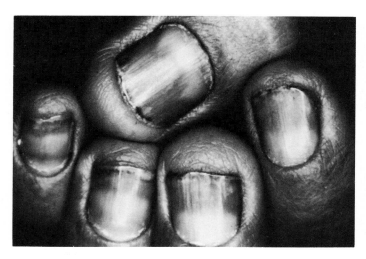

Fig. 36. Changes from paraquat and diquat, appearing like half-and-half nail. (Courtexy Dr. R. Baran)

NOTES

1. Osborne, A.H., Cobden, R., Harvey, J.P., Jr.: Gangrene of infant fingers. *JAMA 221*: 1278-1279, 1972.
2. James, T.: Brittle nails and inquiry into etiology and treatment. *Mediese Bydraes 14*: 9-12, 1968.
3. Stone, O.J., and Maberry, J.D.: Spoon nails and clubbing. *Texas State J. Med. 61*: 620-627, 1965.
4. Samman, P.D. and Johnston, E.N.M. Nail Damage associated with handling of paraquat and dequat. *British Med. J. 1*: 818-819, 1969.
5. Kaufman, J.P. Lichen Striatus with nail involvement. *Cutis 14*:232-233, 1974.
6. Hazelrigg, D.E., Duncan, W.C., and Jarratt, M.: Twenty-nail dystrophy of childhood. *Arch. Derm. 113*: 73-75, 1977.
7. Baran, R. personal communication, 1977.

CHAPTER 18

Hemorrhages

The unique architecture of the nail bed and its supporting dermis results in a series of typical lesions which relate to the disruption of the venules or capillaries in the dermal ridges (see Ch. 1, Figs. 16, 21). Disease or trauma involving blood vessels in an individual or various dermal ridges results in a lesion called splinter hemorrhage. This is seen only in the nail bed area (arrow, Fig. 1; Fig. 2; arrow, Fig. 3). With increased trauma to the nail area, more dermal ridges are involved, resulting in ecchymoses (Fig. 2). Severe trauma causes frank bleeding with extensive hemorrhage. In any event, the size and area involved by the extravasated blood determines the symptomatology.

Originally described by Horder in 1920[1] as a sign of subacute bacterial endocarditis, these line hemorrhages can occur in a series of other diseases (see Table I). The overall incidence in a hospital population is 15–30%; this is remarkably higher than expected (see Table II). Probably an incidence of under 10% is more realistic in United States hospitals. Normal fingers and toes can also present splinter hemorrhages. The thumb and index finger are the most common sites. This is also described in histocytosis-x[2], scurvy, juvenile cirrhosis, anemia, Bechet's, trichinosis, and at high altitudes. The histopathology was described by Alkiewicz in 1933.[3]

Trauma

Everyday trauma may produce hemorrhages of the nail unit. Sports where pivoting quickly and the wearing of tight shoes are involved result in typical hemorrhages of the lateral margins of the nail bed. This is typically seen in tennis (Fig. 4).

Table I

Diseases Associated with Splinter Hemorrhages[1]

	%	*Patients Examined*
Mitral stenosis	86	18
Rheumatic fever (no mitral stenosis)	27	11
Purpura (all causes)	25	4
Arthritis (not rheumatoid)	20	5
Renal disease	20	20
Blood diseases (not purpura)	20	31
Hypertension	18	17
Malignant neoplasm	17	23
Heart disease (not mitral stenosis)	15	80
Pulmonary diseases	12	80
Normal	0	35
Bacterial endocarditis	25	4
Hemodialysis[s]	20	20
Hemachromotosis[a]		

Table II

Overall Incidence of Splinter Hemorrhages in Hospital Population

	Patients Examined	% with Splinter Hemorrhages
Platts & Greaves, 1958[4]	464	17
Gross, 1963[5]	267	19.1
Dowling, 1964[6]	200	60

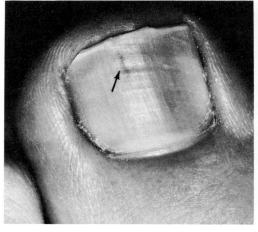

Fig. 1. Splinter hemorrhage (arrow), normal toe.

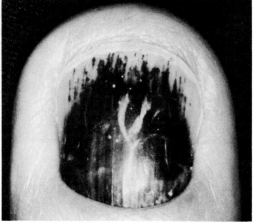

Fig. 2. Three months after car door accident. Note splinter type on periphery.

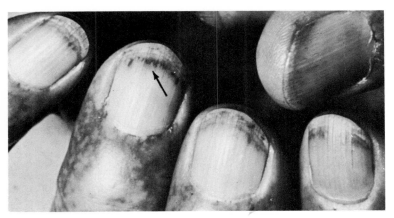

Fig. 3. Distal capillary arc pattern of proximal nail fold commonly accentuated in lupus erythematosus, scleroderma and phototoxic drug eruptions.

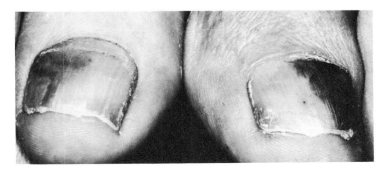

Fig. 4. Tennis buff's toes hemorrhages on lateral aspects of large toes.

NOTES

1. Horder, T.: Splinter hemorrhages of the nail bed. *Brit. Med. J. 2*: 301, 1920.
2. Kahn, G.: Nail involvement in histiocytosis. X. *Arch. Derm. 100*: 699-701, 1969.
3. Alkiewicz, J.: Zur Histopathologie der Hamatome des Menschlichen Nagels. *Arch. Derm. Syph. 168:* 411-419, 1933.
4. Platts, M.M., and Greaves, M.M.: Splinter hemorrhages. *Brit. Med. J. 1*: 143-144, 1958.
5. Gross, N.J.: Clinical significance of splinter hemorrhages. *Brit. Med. J. 40*: 1496-1498, 1963.
6. Dowling, R.H.: Clinical significance of splinter hemorrhages. *Postgrad. Med. J. 40*: 595-600, 1964.
7. Drummond, R.: Splinter hemorrhages at high altitudes. *JAMA 228*: 974, 1974.
8. Blum, M., and Aviram, A.: Splinter hemorrhages in patients receiving regular hemodialysis. *JAMA 239*: p. 47.
9. Lindsay, P.G.: The half-and-half nail. *Arch. Int. Med. 119*: 583-587, 1967.

CHAPTER 19

Pigmentation

Pigmentation of the nail plate is caused by melanin produced by the matrix melanocytes. Melanocytes are seen migrating through the mesenchymal tissues at about 16 to 17 weeks' development in the fetal finger.

The various races naturally have a greater or lesser number of melanocytes in the nail matrix.[1] Pigmentation can be diffuse or bandlike. Diffuse pigmentation usually follows a systemic disease; otherwise, it is rare, even among blacks. Diffuse pigmentation has been described in states where melanocyte stimulating hormone (MSH) is oversecreted, e.g., Addison's, post–Cushing's adrenolectomy, or pituitary tumor.[2] Diffuse melanosis is also seen in patients receiving PUVA (Fig. 8).

BANDLIKE PIGMENTATION

Band pigmentation occurs in 96% of the black population;[3] therefore, it does not represent a source of preoccupation. In Orientals, the incidence of band pigmentation is 11%.[4] In Caucasians, the incidence is about 1%. Pigmented bands have been described in an adrenolectomized patient.[5]

Histopathology of Pigmented Bands

The number of biopsies on pigmented bands is so scanty and the technical problems in processing these biopsies so great that very little can be generalized. In blacks with pigmented bands that widened (three biopsies), the histopathology is melanocytic hyperplaseia. There is no atypia. In Caucasians (four biopsies), the same was found. One cannot generalize from this experience. For the present, to be conservative seems the best policy: in non-blacks, remove locally matrix melanocytes by simple excision; in blacks, do nothing but observe. See chapter 29–Melanocytic Lesions.

PIGMENTATION OF NAIL AND ORAL MUCOSA (Longitudinal Bonds)

Pigmentation of the nail matrix occurs associated with macular pigmentation of the oral mucosa (lips, etc). First described by Lauggier and Hunziker,[22] and was recently reassessed by Baran.[23]

DIFFERENTIATION OF EXTERNAL AND INTERNAL NAIL PIGMENTATION

Other pigmentations are also seen in and on the nail. To make the differentiation between "on" (externally deposited pigments) and "in" (internally deposited pigments), it is crucial to see the most proximal border's shape (opposite the distal free edge). If the pigmentation follows the proximal nail fold and the lateral nail fold shapes (as in Fig. 6), then it is caused by external sources (in this case, by Esoterica cream, but also commonly by numerous hair-darkening agents).

A shape following the shape of the lunula (as seen in Wilson's disease or argyria) is characteristically internally produced as seen in Fig. 7, Chemotherapy.

Table I lists common causes of nail pigmentation.

NAIL PLATE CHANGES SECONDARY TO COSMETICS

Nail polish may cause the surface of the nail to take on a whitish, blotchy appearance, usually ill-defined so that one cannot appreciate the configuration of the PNF. The nail bed is not involved as it was twenty years ago, since most of the solvents that "went through" the nail plate have been removed from the market. Occasionally, a subungual discoloration is seen with frosted nail polish.

ULTRAVIOLET LIGHT A AND THE NAIL PLATE

Generalized nail bed pigmentation can be seen in PUVA therapy, especially in the nail bed (Fig. 8). UV-A must go through the translucent nail plate. Where are the melanocytes in the nail bed to produce such a hyperpigmentation?

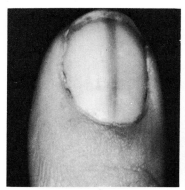 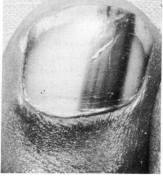 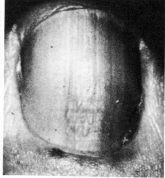

Fig. 1. Pigmented band in 12-year-old boy. Rare.

Fig. 2. Pigmented band in black female. Common.

Fig. 3. Very wide pigmented band in Caucasian male who also had Addison's disease. Band widened over past four years.

Table I

Nail Various Colors and Their Cause

Nail Color	Cause	Deposit Location
Black	Peutz-Jeghers syndrome	Nail bed, matrix
Black	Vitamin B$_{12}$ deficiency[6]	Nail bed, matrix
Black	Pinta[7]	Nail bed
Black	Ammoniated mercuric sulfide[8,9]	Nail plate surface
Black	Hair dyes	Nail plate surface
Black	Post-irradiation[10]	Matrix, nail plate
Black streak	Melanocytic hyperplasia	Matrix, nail plate
Black streak	Malignant melanoma	Matrix, nail plate
Gray-black	Silver salts[11]	Lunula
Gray-black	Malignant melanoma	Matrix, nail plate
Dark gray	Phenolphthalein[12]	Lunula
Gray	Mercuric chloride[13]	Nail plate surface
Brown-black	Fungus	Nail plate
Brown-black	Photographic developer	Nail plate surface
Brown	Vitiligo	Nail bed
Red-brown	Resorcin, nail lacquer[14]	Nail plate surface
Blue-brown	Chloroquine-aralen[15]	Nail bed, nail plate
Blue-brown	Quinacrine-atabrine[16,17]	Nail bed, nail plate
Blue-brown	Amodiaquine-camoquin[18]	Nail bed, nail plate
Blue-brown	Wilson's disease[19]	Lunula
Green	Pseudomonas	Nail plate
Yellow	Yellow nail syndrome	Nail plate
White bands	Arsenic-Mee's lines[20,21]	Nail plate

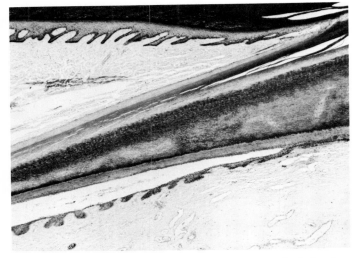

Fig. 4. Photomicrograph of biopsy taken from finger in Fig. 1, showing proximal nail fold (PNF), nail plate (NP) and matrix (M). Silver H&E X120..

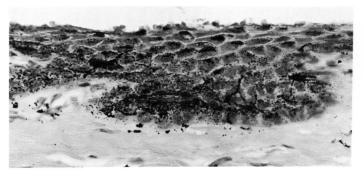

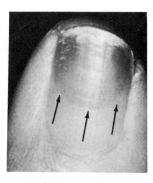

Fig. 5. Photomicrograph at higher magnification of arrow in Fig. 4, showing abundant normal-appearing melanocytes in matrix. (Silver X800)

Fig. 6. Pigmented pattern is that of proximal nail fold. Hallmark of pigmentation due to topical agents. Most common is Esoterica cream to remove pigment.

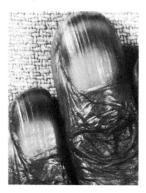

Fig. 7. Lunula pattern is hallmark of systemic causes for pigmentation; Dauteromycin therapy for GYN malignancy.

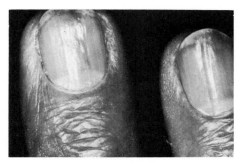

Fig. 8. Diffuse hyperpigmentation of nail bed seen in patient treated with PUVA for psoriasis. Pigmentation reduces as time without PUVA goes on.

NOTES

1. Monash, S.: Normal pigmentation in the nails of the Negro. *Arch. Derm. Syph. 25*: 876-881, 1932.
2. Lerner, A.B., and McGuire, J.S.: Melanocyte-stimulating hormone and adrenocorticotrophic hormone; their relation to pigmentation. *New Eng. J. Med. 270*: 539-546, 1964.
3. Leyden, J.J., Spott, D.A., and Goldschmidt, P.: Diffuse and banded melanin pigmentation. *Arch. Derm. 105*: 548-550, 1972.
4. Kawamura, T., et al: On pigmentation longitudinalis striata unguim. *Jap. J. Derm. 68*: 10, 1958.
5. Bondy, P.K., and Harwick, H.J.: Longitudinal banded pigmentation of nails following adrenalectomy for Cushing's syndrome. *New Eng. J. Med. 281*: 1056-1058, 1969.
6. Baker, S.J., Ignatius, M., Johnson, S., and Vaish, S.K.: Hyperpigmentation of skin. *Brit. Med. J. 5347*: 1713-1715, 1963.
7. Medina, R.: El carate en Venezuela. *Derm. Venezolana 3*: 160-230, 1963.
8. John, F.: Ueber die Schwarzfarbung tierischen und menschlicher Hornsubstanz nach Impragnation mit Quecksilberlosungen und den Einfluss des Sonnenlichtes auf den Ablauf der ursächlichen chemischen Umsetzung, *Derm. Wschr. 100*: 728, 1935.

9. Butterworth, T., and Strean, L.P.: Mercurial pigmentation of nails. *Arch. Derm. 88*: 55-57, 1963.
10. Shelly, W.B., Rawnsley, H.M., and Pillsbury, D.M.: Postirradiation melanonychia. *Arch. Derm. 90*: 174-176, 1964.
11. Koplon, B.S.: Azure lunulae due to argyria. *Arch. Derm. 94*: 333-334, 1966.
12. Campbell, G.S.: Peculiar pigmentation following the use of a purgative containing phenolphthalein. *Brit J. Derm. 43*: 186-187, 1931.
13. Callaway, J.L.: Transient discoloration of the nails due to mercury bichloride. *Arch. Derm. 36*: 62-64, 1937.
14. Loveman, A.B., and Fliegelman, M.T.: Discoloration of the nails. *Arch. Derm. 72*: 153-156, 1955.
15. Tuffanelli, D., Abraham, R.K., and Dubois, E.I.: Pigmentation from antimalarial therapy. *Arch. Derm. 88*: 419-426, 1963.
16. Kierland, R.R., Shard, C., Mason, H.L., and Lobitz, W.C.: Fluorescence of nails from quinacrine hydrochloride. *JAMA 131*: 809-810, 1946.
17. Barr, J.F.: Subungual pigmentation following prolonged atabrine therapy. *US Naval Med. Bull. 43*: 929, 1944.
18. Maguire, A.: Amodiaquine hydrochloride, corneal deposits and pigmented palate and nails after treatment of chronic discoid lupus erythematosus. *Lancet 1*: 667, 1962.
19. Bearn, A.G., and McKuscik, V.A. Azure lunulae—an unsual change in the fingernails in two patients with hepatolenticular degeneration (Wilson's disease). *JAMA 166*: 903-906, 1958.
20. Althausen, T.L., and Gunther, L.: Acute arsenic poisoning. *JAMA 92*: 2002-2006, 1929.
21. Simmons, G.P.: Beginning, duration and course of action of arsenic on nails. Abstract, *JAMA 94*, 1937.
22. Laugier, P., and Hunziker, N.: Pigmentation melanique lenticulaire essentielle de la muqueuse jugaie et des levres. *Arch. Dermatol. et Syph. 26*: 391-399, 1970.
23. Baran, R.: Longitudinal melanotic streaks as a clue to Laugier-Hunziker Syndrome. *Arch. Dermatol. 115*: 1448-1449, 1979.

CHAPTER 20

Leukonychia

The white (opaque) appearance of any part or of all the nail plate is termed leukonychia. Although it was described in the early 1880's, Mitchell[1] has written the most comprehensive clinical report on the fate of a leukonychic spot. Mitchell observed 105 spots and found that only 45 reached the free edge; of those, the surface area diminished considerably in their distal migrations.

Leukonychias are divided into acquired and congenital. Congenital leukonchia can occur as an isolated phenomenon or can exist with koilonychia and/or with hearing loss (Fig. 2). Acquired leukonychia has been described following numerable circumstances and events. Table I shows reported events associated with leukonychia. The shapes that leukonychias assume are also a favorite subject for investigation: whole nails, bands (Figs. 3, 4), fragments, dots, etc.

Histology

In 1900, Heidingsfeld[2] described the pathology of a leukonychia as a focus of retained nuclei (parakeratosis) in the nail plate (Fig. 1). Later, Ackriewicz[3] (1935) added that there were also large brownish granules which, by all his tests of that time, were not keratonyalin in nature but rather took silver stains and resembled melanin. These he termed leucomelanin granules.

No new evidence on the nature of these granules exists today. Another possibility is that the brownish granules are due to formalin fixation.

Table I

Leukonychias

CONGENITAL

1. Isolated
2. Associated with koilonychia (spooning)
3. Associated with deafness
4. Leukonychia totalis, multiple sebaceous cysts, renal calculi[4]

ACQUIRED

1. Addison's disease
2. Antimetabolite therapy
3. Arsenic toxicity (Mee's lines)
4. Cardiac insufficiency
5. Fluorosis
6. Exfoliative dermatitis
7. Hodgkin's disease
8. Infectious fevers (Reil's Lines)
9. Malaria
10. Menstrual cycle
12. Myocardial infarction
13. Leprosy
14. Occupational
15. Pellagra
16. Pneumonia
17. Sickle cell anemia
18. Thallium toxicity
19. TBC
20. Trichinosis
21. Zinc deficiency
22. Fungal infections (proximal subungual)
23. Zoster

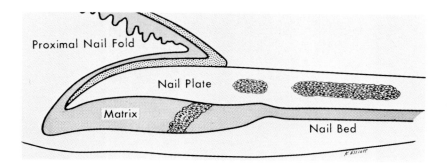

Fig. 1. Diagrammatic drawing of pathogenesis of white appearance of nail. Parakeratotic onychocytes with or without "grains" result in a diffusion of light going through that comes off "white."

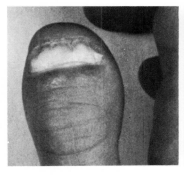 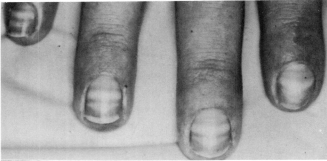

Fig. 2. Leukonychia, koilonychia and deafness. Hereditary.

Fig. 3. Acquired leukonychial bands. Antimetabolyte treatment for leukemia. (Courtesy Dr. A. Hernandez).

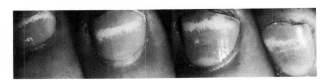

Fig. 4. Acquired leukonychial bands. Cause unknown.

NOTES

1. Mitchell, J.C.: A clinical study of leukonychia. *Brit. J. Derm. 65*: 14-130, 1953.
2. Heidingsfeld, M.L.: The pathology of leukonychia. *J. Cutan. Dis. 18*: 490, 1900.
3. Alkiewicz, J.: Clinical & histopathologic studies on leukonychia. *Przegl. Dermat. 30*: 109-144, 1935.
4. Bushkell, L.L., and Gorlin, R.J.: Leukonychia totalis, multiple sebaceous cysts, renal calculi[4] *Arch. Derm. 111*: 899-901, 1975.

CHAPTER 21

Scabies Keratotic (Norwegian)

This fascinating disease is produced by the scabetic mite (sarcoptes scabie; hominis) (Fig. 5) living on the surface of a patient who has an as yet unknown defect in his cellular immunity mechanism. These hosts may be mentally retarded (Fig. 1, shown with her mother) or physically debilitated.

In keratotic scabies, the mite is present in incredibly high numbers. (Ordinary scabies is said to have no more than 20 mites over all the body.). Clinically, keratotic areas may be present in the scalp, the face (never in regular scabies), palms (Fig. 2) and soles.

The mite destroys the nail from the surface down (Fig. 3, 4). Complete destruction of the nail plate may occur; usually, no great pruritis is present (variable).

Treatment

The treatment is an anti-scabicide.

Nail changes similar to nail keratotic scabies are also seen in chronic granulomatous disease of childhood.

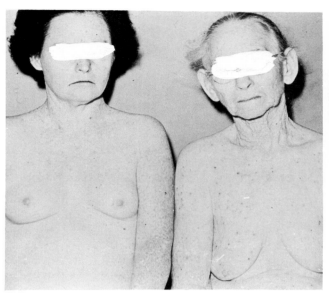

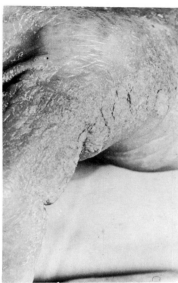

Fig. 1. Mother and daughter with scabies. Mother has normal type; daughter with Downs syndrome has keratotic or Norwegian type.

Fig. 2. Norwegian or keratotic scabies may occur on hands, feet and face.

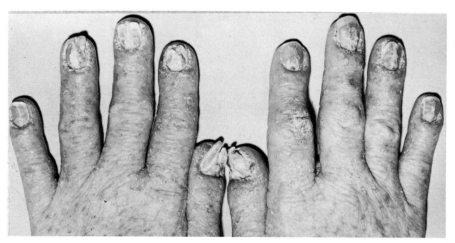

Fig. 3. Massive dystrophy of nail plate. Myriads of acari are present in nails. Appearance similar to chronic mucocutaneous.

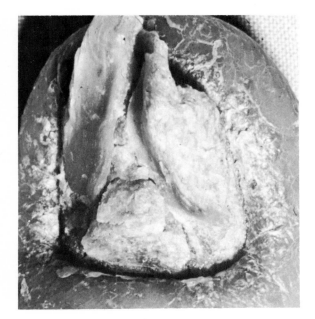

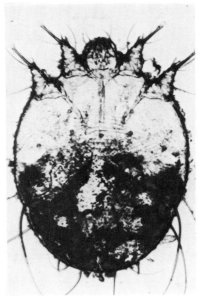

Fig. 4. Nail plate destruction.

Fig. 5. Sarcoptes scabiei.

CHAPTER 22

Nail Signs as Manifestations of Systemic Diseases

Generally, nail signs in relation to systemic disease have been greatly overrated. Normally, nail signs serve more as a confirmation of systemic disease than as a clue leading to early diagnosis. There are, however, some nail signs that begin earlier than the signs and symptoms of the underlying disease. Table I describes these as diagnostic and Table II as associated with systemic disease. In particular, Basex's acrokeratoses seems to be a unique indication of malignancy for months preceding the overt symptoms.

Table II summarizes diseases in which nail changes are not early and usually are an adjunct to diagnosis by other means.

Table III summarizes diseases in which nail changes may occur randomly and are of no diagnostic value.

Table I
Nail Unit Signs Diagnostic of Underlying Disease

Psoriasiform changes on tip of finger and nail unit (sudden onset without familial history)	Underlying neoplastic disease (Basex paraneoplastic acrokeratose)
Clubbing (see Ch. XXIII)	Pulmonary
Yellow nail not growing (yellow nail syndrome; see Ch. XXIV)	Pulmonary disease, edema and effusions
Pterygium inversus[6] unguis (acquired)	Scleroderma

Table II

Nail Unit Signs Associated With and Present in Systemic Disease

Splinter hemorrhages in nail bed	See Ch. 18, Table II
Numerous and abnormal capillary loops in proximal nail fold	Lupus erythematosus, dermatomysitis, cystic fibrosis, diabetes mellitus, congenital heart disease, mongolism, schizophrenia
Spoon nails (koilonychia)	Sideropenic dysphagia (Plummer-Vinson or Paterson-Kelly syndrome), anemia, idiopathic hemochromatosis
Poikilodermatous skin of knuckle and proximal nail fold	Dermatomyositis
Onycholysis	Thyroid, Bantu porphyria, erythropoetic protoporphyria, porphyria cutanea tarda, phototoxic drug eruption, pellagra
Half-white/half-red nail bed	Renal disease
Hyperpigmentation of nail bed	Increased MSH, Addison's disease (see Ch. 19)
Massive reddish paronychial infiltrates with atrophy of nail plate	Histiocytosis-X may also have scalp involvement. Pulmonary symptoms decreased breathing "reserve"

Table III

Systemic Disease with Random Nail Localization

Alopecia mucinosa[27]
Discoid lupus erythematosus
Metastic disease (see Ch. 26)
Mycosis fungoides (see Ch. 26)
Pemphigoid
Pemphigus[22,23]
Pityriasis rosea[24]
Sarcoid
Syphilis
Lichen striatus[25]
Toxic epidermal necrolysis[26]
(Lyell syndrome)

ACRAL-PSORIASIFORM PREMALIGNANT DERMATOSES OF BASEX

This remarkable syndrome consists of an acute psoriasiform eruption in the acral parts (hands, feet, nose and ears) (Figs. 1–5) of patients who have never had a family history of psoriasis. First described by Basex in 1965[1] and reviewed by Baran in 1978,[2] it presents another example of a skin and nail symptom complex as the result of a neoplasm (usually upper gastrointestinal tract or respiratory tract) which precedes the symptomatology of the neoplasm by months and which promptly disappears after the removal of the neoplasm. Braverman[3] in his book *Cutaneous Manifestation of Systemic Disease* describes two patients with psoriasifrom eruptions who eventually developed neoplasms. Recently, Samitz[4] described psoriasiform changes in the cuticle of patients with dermatomyositis who may have had or developed neoplasms. These psoriasiform changes could be an expansion of Basex. Recently, Shupack and associates[5] have described a female who developed psoriasiform skin and nail changes four years prior to the discovery of her malignant glucogonoma.

PTERYGIUM INVERSUM UNGUIS (ACQUIRED)

This is truly a helpful sign toward diagnosing scleroderma and may occur at the same time the disease becomes symptomatic. The volar skin near the hyponychium becomes atrophic secondary to vascular occlusion (slow). These ischemic areas may involve one-half the volar aspect of the entire hyponychium. This was excellently demonstrated by Patterson (1978).[6]

CLUBBING

See Chapter 23.

YELLOW NAIL SYNDROME

See Chapter 24.

SPLINTER HEMORRHAGES

See Chapter 18.

CAPILLARY LOOPS IN THE PROXIMAL NAIL FOLD

Normally, the skin of the proximal nail fold is a continuation of dorsum digit skin but has adapted to become fingertip skin in that: (1) it is shaped like a wedge or apex, (2) it is devoid of hair follicles and (3) it is very thin at the apex of the wedge, thus allowing a better visualization of the underlying capillary and venule loops (Fig. 12). These loops have been described by many investigators as hallmark signs of underlying systemic disease.[29] Usually, this is a phenomenon seen in fingers. These capillary loops occur normally but are few in number. An excessive number of these vascular loops and their occurrence in most fingers are associated with so-called lupus erythematosus;[7] they have also been described in dermatomyositis,[8] cystic fibrosis,[8] congenital heart disease, mongolism,[8] schizophrenia,[9] and diabetes mellitus.[10]

KOILONYCHIA (SPOON NAILS)

This nail sign[11] accompanies the clinical syndrome termed sideropenic dysphagia (Plummer-Vinson or Paterson-Kelly syndrome). It occurs in women in the forty- to fifty-year-old age group who also have difficulty in swallowing, fatigability, and anemia. An upper-tract alimentary carcinoma is associated as well. Koilonychias are seen in approximately 50% of idiopathic hemochromatoses[12] and in iron-deficient anemics.

POIKILODERMATOUS SKIN

This complex sign of various shades of pink and red skin associated with slight atrophy and telangiectasia is seen in dermatomyositis (Fig. 14). Characteristically on the proximal nail fold and over the knuckle areas sparing the outer knuckle skin, this poikilodermatous skin appears during the active phases of the disease and may disappear after correction of the disease. Lichenification of knuckle skin can be occupationally related; this should not be confused with poikiloderma of these areas. In poikiloderma of the knuckles, a lichenification may occur resulting in a papule as first described by Grotton in dermatomyositis.

ONYCHOLYSIS

Onycholysis is believed to be a common sign of hyperthyroid, but only one study (Caravati and associates[14]) reported 5.2% of onycholytic nails in 120 thyroid patients.

BANTU PORPHYRIA[28]

This unique clinical syndrome consists of skin which blisters when exposed to the sun, darkening face and hands, and nail dystrophy. The nail dystrophy begins with blistering of the nail bed and consequent uplifting of the nail plate. The nail plate softens, leading to nail plate damage and eventual dystrophy.

ERYTHROPOETIC PROTOPORPHYRIA

Schmidt and co-workers[15] studied a large group of patients with EPP. The predominant nail lesion was onycholysis, probably a blister in the nail bed. The fingertips were painful. One case suddenly presented with total leukonychia.

GASTROINTESTINAL POLYPOSIS, PROTEIN-LOSING ENTEROPATHY, ABNORMAL SKIN PIGMENTATION AND LOSS OF HAIR AND NAILS (CRONKHITE-CANADA SYNDROME)

Described in 1955,[16] the skin pigmentation is melanotic, the nail dystrophy is atrophy and the intestinal polyposis benign.

THE HALF-AND-HALF NAIL

This syndrome was originally described by Bean[17] and further studied by Lindsay.[18] Among 24 patients who were azotemic, 21 had the distal portion of their fingernails reddish to brown in color.

HEPATOLENTICULAR DEGENERATION (WILSON'S DISEASE)

Bluish lunula are characteristic of this syndrome (Wilson's disease).

FEMINIZATION IN MALES

Thickening of nail plates was reported in two patients: one secondary to hypopituitarism with feminine genotype;[19] the second after accidental loss of the testes.[20]

MULTICENTRIC RETICULOHISTIOCYTOSIS

Accordion-shaped fingers and short nail plates are characteristic of this condition.[21]

HISTIOCYTOSIS-X[30]

See chapter on malignancies and nail.

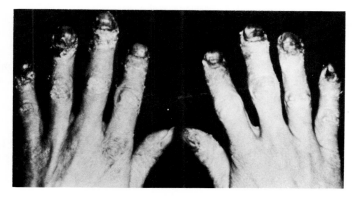

Fig. 1. Basex malignant psoriasiform acrokeratosis. Psoriasiform dermatitis around fingernails. (Courtesy Dr. Basex.)

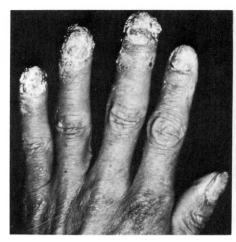

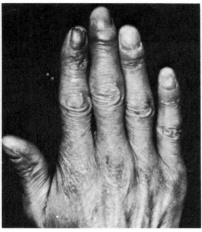

Fig. 2. Basex malignant psoriasiform acro-keratosis. Skin and nail signs months before upper GI neoplasm. (Courtesy Dr. Basex.)

Fig. 3. Patient in Fig. 2, after removal of GI neoplasm. (Courtesy Dr. Basex.)

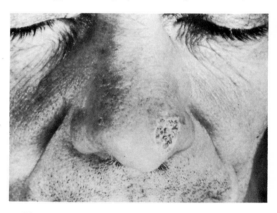

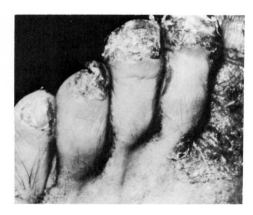

Fig. 4. Same patient showing eczematous-scaly plaque on acral (nose) area. (Courtesy Dr. Basex.)

Fig. 5. Feet of same patient. (Courtesy Dr. Basex.)

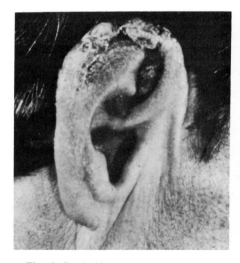

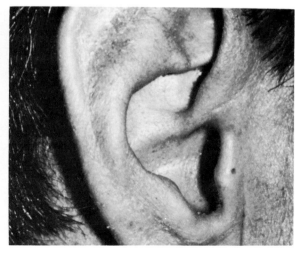

Fig. 6. Psoriasiform plaque, same patient. (Courtesy Dr. Basex.)

Fig. 7. Ear cleared after surgical removal of GI lesions. (Courtesy Dr. Basex.)

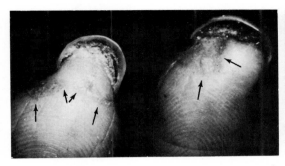

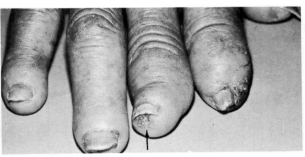

Fig. 8. Scleroderma. Ischemic tip of digit, also called acquired pterygium inversum unguis. (Courtesy Dr. Basex.)

Fig. 9. Scleroderma, more severe ischemic lesion, tips of index and middle finger.

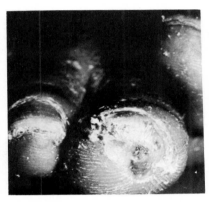

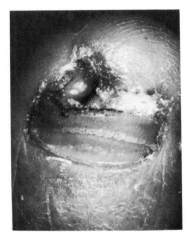

Fig. 10. Close-up, tip of index finger in patient in Fig. 9, showing severe changes similar to changes (more subtle) in Fig. 8.

Fig. 11. Ischemic ulceration of nail bed in artheriosclerosis–diabetes mellitus patient. Base of ulcer is phalanx.

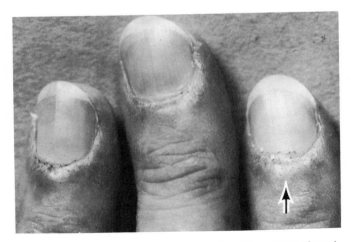

Fig. 12. Lupus erythematosus, accentuated capillary plexus of proximal nail fold (arrow).

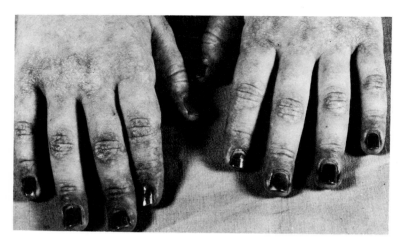

Fig. 13. Dermatolyositis. Poikilodermatous changes over knuckle areas, fine papules also present. (Dermatology, University of Miami.)

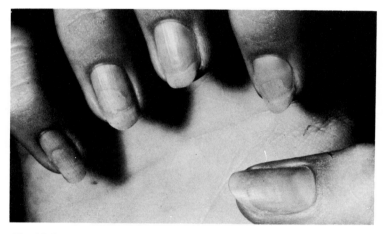

Fig. 14. Dermatomyositis. Papules on knuckle areas; described first by Grokot. (University of Miami, Derm.)

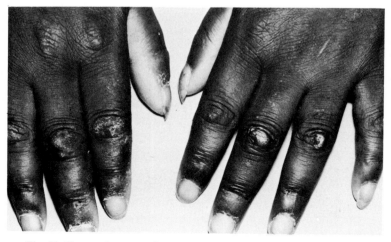

Fig. 15. Phototoxic tetracycline reactions, onycholysis.

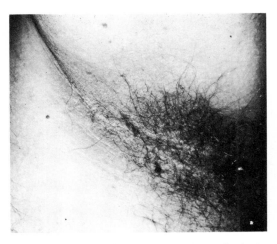

Fig. 16. Addison's disease. Patient with acanthosis nigricans and marked hyperpigmentation.

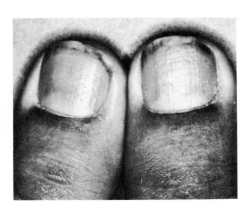

Fig. 17. Patient in Fig. 16. Hyperpigmentation of proximal nail fold, fine pitting of nail plate surface.

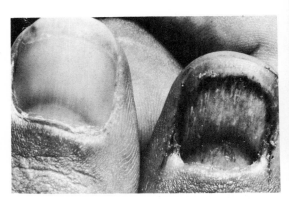

Fig. 18. Wilson's disease (hepatolenticular degeneration). Thumb on left showing blue haze of lunula. Thumb on right with nail plate off showing not blue color but increased vascular network around lunula. (University of Miami, Department of Dermatology)

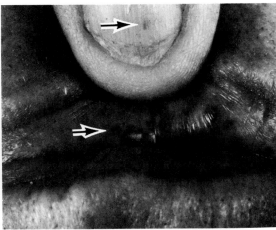

Fig. 19. Hereditary hemorrhagic telangectasia; Osler-Rendu-Welser. Nail bed (arrow) and lips. (Department of Dermatology, University of Miami.)

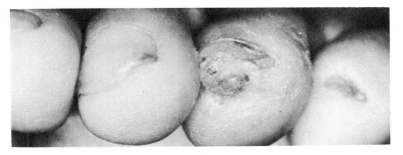

Fig. 20. Onycholymadesis: systemic corticosteroids for treatment of severe drug eruption.

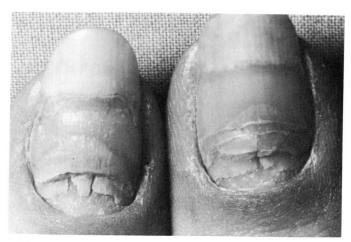

Fig. 21. Sarcoidosis: subungual papule. (Department of Dermatology, University of Miami.)

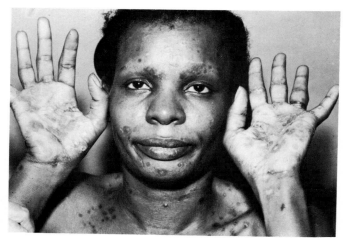

Fig. 22. Secondary syphilis. (University of Miami, Department of Dermatology.)

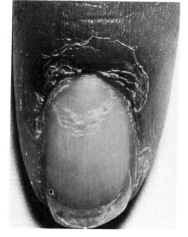

Fig. 23. Secondary syphilis: papule on PNF affecting proximal matrix. (University of Miami, Department of Dermatology.)

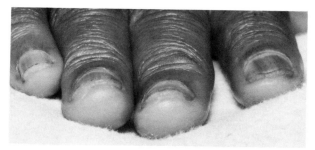

Fig. 24. Hypothyroidism: acquired, thickened nail bed and hyponychium(?). (Department of Dermatology, University of Miami.)

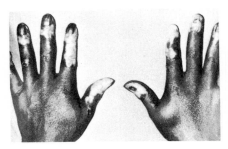

Fig. 25. Discoid lupus erythematosus. (Courtesy Dr. R. Caputo.)

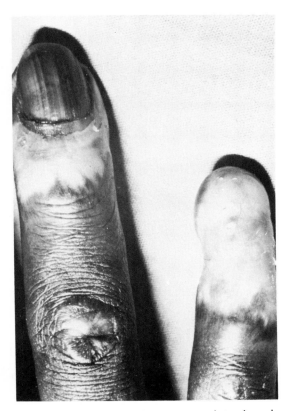

Fig. 26. Discoid lupus erythematosus: total atrophy and scarring. (Courtesy Dr. R. Caputo.)

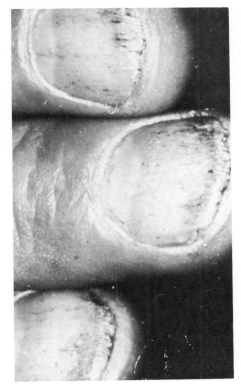

Fig. 27. Splinter hemorrhages in alopecia mucinosa.

NOTES

1. Basex, A., Salvador R., Dupre, A., and Christol B.: Syndrome paraneoplasique a type d'hyperkeratose des extremites. Guerison apres traitement de l'epithelioma larynge. *Bull. Soc. Fr. Der. et Syph.* *72*: 182, 1965.

2. Baran, R.: Basex's acrokeratose neoplastique. *Arch. Derm.* *117*: 1613, 1977.

3. Braverman, I.M.: *Skin Signs of Systemic Disease.* Philadelphia: W.B. Saunders, 1970, p. 169.

4. Samitz, M.H.: Cuticular changes in dermatomyositis. *Arch. Derm.* *110*: 865, 1974.

5. Shupack, J.L., Beczeller, P.H., and Stevens, D.M. The Glucagonoma Syndrome. *J. Dermatol. Surg. Oncol.* *4*: 242-247, 1978.

6. Patterson, J.W.: Pterygium inversum unguis. A nail sign in scleroderma. *Arch. Derm.* *113*: 1421, 1977.

7. Ross, J.B.: Nail fold capillaroscopy—a useful aid in the diagnosis of collagen vascular diseases. *J. Invest. Derm.* *47*: 282-285, 1966.

8. Higashino, S.M., and Moss, A.J.: Capillary microscopy, *Amer. J. Dis. Child 113*: 439-443, 1967.

9. Marico, H.R.: Association of a clearly visible subpapillary plexus with other peculiarities of the nailfold skin in some schizophrenic patients. *Dermatologica 138*: 148-154, 1969.

10. Landau, J., and Davis, E.: The small blood-vessels of the conjunctiva and nailbed in diabetes mellitus. *Lancet*: 731-734, 1960.

11. Waldenstrom, J.: Iron and epithelium. Some clinical observations. *Acta Med. Scand.* (Suppl.), *90*: 380-397, 1938.

12. Chevrant -Breton, J., Simons, M., Bourel, M., and Ferrand, B.: Cutaneous manifestations of idiopathic hemochromatosis. *Arch. Derm. 113*: 161-165, 1977.

13. Rosenbaum, E., and Leonard, J.W.: Nutritional iron deficiency anemia in an adult male. *Ann. Internal Med. 60*: 683-688, 1964.

14. Caravati, J.C., Richardson, D.R., Wood, B.T., and Cawley, E.P.: Cutaneous manifestations of hyperthyroid disease. *Southern Med. J. 62*: 1127-1130, 1969.

15. Schmidt, H., Snitker, G., Thomsen, K., and Lintrup, J.: Erythopoetic protoporphyria. *Arch. Derm, 110*: 58-64, 1974.

16. Cronkhite, L.W., Jr., and Canada, W.J.: Generalized gastrointestinal polyposis. *N. Eng. J. Med. 252*: 1011-1015, 1955.

17. Bean, W.B.: Half-and-half nail. *Trans. Amer. Clin. Climat. Assoc. 74*: 152-167, 1963.

18. Lindsay, P.G.: The half-and-half nail. *Arch. Int. Med. 119*: 583-587, 1967.

19. Hollander, L.: Onychauxis due to hypopiturtarism. *Arch. Derm. Syph. 3*: 35-43, 1920.

20. Lisser, H.: Onychauxis in a eunuchoid. *Arch. Derm. Syph. 7*: 180-182, 1924.

21. Barrow, M.V.: The nails in multicentric reticulohistiocytosis. *Arch. Derm. 95*, 1967.

22. Stone, O.J., and Mullins, F.J.: Vegetative lesions in Pemphigus. *Dermatologia Internationalis 5*: 137-140, 1966.

23. Baumal, A., and Rovinson, M.J. Nail bed involvement in pemphigus vulgaris. *Arch. Derm. 107*: 751, 1973.

24. Silvers, S.H., and Glickman, F.: Ptyriasis Rosea followed by nail dystrophy. *Arch. Derm. 90*: 31, 1964.

25. Kaufman, J.P.: Lichen striatus with nail involvement. *Cutis 14*: 232-233, 1974.

26. Jaramillo, O., Soto, M., Lara, F., and Rodriguez, O. Syndrome de Lyell. *Arta Medica Cost. 16*: 215-233, 1973.

27. Lapiere, S., Castermans, E. and Pierard, E. Mucinose folliculaire et ungueale generalisee. *Soc. Fran. Dermat. et Syph. 9*: 235, 1972.

28. Gelfand, M., and Mitchell, J.D.: Bantu porphyria. *Trans. Royal Soc. Trop. Med. Hyg. 51*: 62-68, 1957.

29. Zimmer, J.G., and Demis, D.J.: Studies on the microcirculation in disease. *J. Invest. Derm. 39*: 501-509, 1962.

30. Kahn, G. Nail Involvement in Histocytosis-X. *Arch. Derm. 100*: 699-701, 1969.

CHAPTER 23

Clubbing of the Fingers

Synonyms for this condition are hippocratic nails, hippocratic fingers, acropachy, dysacromelia, trommelschlagelfinger.

Since Aristotle's time, clubbing of the fingers has been recognized as an early sign of underlying disease; however, idiopathic clubbing may occur without underlying pulmonary or other visceral disease (see Tables I, II).

Anatomic considerations in making a diagnosis of clubbing include:

1. Bulbous, fusiform enlargement of the distal portion of the fingers and toes.

2. Abnormal "profile sign"[1] or increase in the normal "hyponychial angle"[2] The latter, recently described, actually attempts to quantitate Lovibond's profile sign angle.

3. No abnormality of underlying phalanx.

4. A noticeable mobility of the matrix as one pushes down and away from the distal interphalangeal joint. This mobility is due to an increase (hyperplasia) in the fibrovascular tissues[3] between the matrix and the phalanx, producing the fusiform enlargement and the abnormal profile sign.

IDIOPATHIC CLUBBING

Idiopathic and hereditary clubbing[4] may be inherited as a simple Mendelian dominant or as an autosomal dominant sex-limited trait with variable penetrance. The abnormality has an insidious onset, usually starting after puberty. It affects both fingernails and toenails (Fig. 1, 2). Pachydermoperiostosis[5,6] is included in this group since the forme fruste may exhibit simple clubbing and cutis gyrata.

ACQUIRED OR SECONDARY CLUBBING

This type of clubbing may be symmetrical, unilateral or digital.[7-10] Symmetrical clubbing may occur in association with infectious, noninfectious, neoplastic, pulmonary, bronchial and mediastinal disease. Commonly associated with lung carcinoma, it also occurs with cyanotic cardiovascular disease, hepatic cirrhosis, chronic diarrheal disease and other miscellaneous conditions. Unilateral and unidigital clubbing always are seen in relation to localized vascular lesions, e.g., aneurysm, arteriovenous fistula. Reports indicate that the earliest a malignancy has been diagnosed after the onset of clubbing is at 18 months.

Table I
Classification of Digital Clubbing

Idiopathic	Secondary
Hereditary (simple)	Associated with vascular abnormality (local)
Pachydermoperiostosis	Associated with systemic diseases
Forme fruste complete	Associated with hypertrophic osteoarthropathy and periostosis

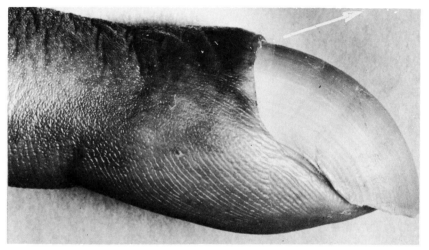

Fig. 1. Clubbed finger showing Lovigond's angle greater than 180 . (See Chapter I, Fig. 2.)

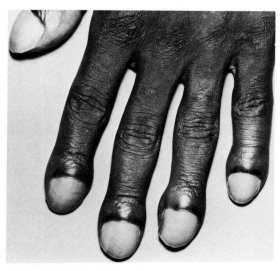

Fig. 2. Idiopathic clubbing.

Table II
Characteristics of Digital Clubbing

Factor	Hereditary (simple)	Idiopathic Pachydermoperiostosis (complete syndrome)	Simple	Secondary Clubbing & Hypertrophic Osteoarthropathy
History	Gradual onset; family history	Onset after puberty	Gradual or sudden onset; no family history	Gradual onset
Symptoms	None	None	None	Pain
Sex	Equal	Males	Equal	Mostly males
Skin	Normal	Cutis gyrata, seborrhea	Normal	Normal
Bones	Normal	No definite radiolucent line between periosteal new bone and thickened cortex	Normal	Definite radiolucent line between periosteal new bone and thickened cortex
Joints	Normal	Occasional abnormalities	Normal	Chronic painful synovitis
Physiologic response of blood vessels in bulbous tip (blood flow)	Normal	Decreased	Increased	Increased

Table III

Acquired Diseases Resulting in Clubbing[s]

ACQUIRED

PULMONARY

1. Neoplasms of lung
2. Bronchitis, emphysema, lung abscess, cyst, tuberculosis, pulmonary fibrosis, blastomycosis, acute pneumonia, pulmonary endarteritis, chronic passive congestion
3. Mediastinal-fibrosarcoma, meso-endothelioma, Hodgkin's disease, lyphoma, pseudo-tumor (dilation of esophagus)
4. Metastatic neoplasm (fibrosarcoma, giant cell tumor)

CARDIOVASCULAR

1. Congenital heart disease (cyanotic)
2. Subacute bacterial endocarditis
3. Congestive heart failure
4. Chronic myelogenous leukemia
5. Myxoid tumor
6. Acyanotic congenital heart diseases (rare)

HEPATIC

1. Cirrhosis (cholangiolitic, malarial, hemochromatotic)
2. Portal cirrhosis, secondary amyloidosis

GASTROINTESTINAL

1. Chronic diarrhea, sprue
2. Ulcerative colitis
3. Neoplasms
4. Ascaris

RENAL—CHRONIC PYELONEPHRITIS (rare)

TOXIC

Phosphorus, arsenic, alcohol, mercury, beryllium, reduced ferritin

MISCELLANEOUS (rare)

Syphilis, syringomyelia, Maffucci's syndrome, congenital dysplasia, angiectasis, chronic familial neutropenia, post-thyroidectomy, myxedema, cretinism, primary polycythemia, leprosy, rheumatic fever, Raynaud's disease, scleroderma, acrocyanosis, chilblains, Kaposi's sarcoma

UNILATERAL OR UNIDIGITAL

Areterial aneurysm (aortic, axillary)
Brachial ateriovenous fistula
Subluxation of shoulder
Pancoast tumors
Erythromelalgia
Lymphangitis
Median nerve injury
Local trauma
Felon
Tophaceous gout
Sarcoidosis

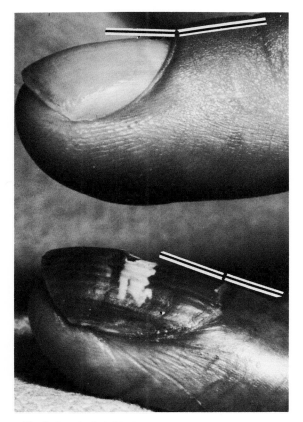

Fig. 3. Acquired clubbed finger, secondary to pulmonary neoplasm

NOTES

1. Lovibond, J. L.: Diagnosis of clubbed fingers, *Lancet 1*:363-364, 1938.
2. Regan, G. M., Tagg, B., and Thomson, M. L.: Subjective assessment and objective measurement of finger clubbing, *Lancet 1*:530-532, 1967.
3. Bigler, F. C.: The morphology of clubbing, *Amer J Path 34*: 237-261, 1958.
4. Fischer, D. S., Singer, D. H., and Feldman, S. M.: Clubbing: A review with emphasis on hereditary acropachy, *Medicine 43*:459-479, 1964.
5. Hambrick, G. W., Jr., and Carter, D. M.: Pachydermoperiostosis, *Arch Derm 94*:594-608, 1966.
6. Rimoin, D. L.: Pachydermoperiostosis (idiopathic clubbing and periostosis), *New Eng J. Med 272*:923-931, 1965.
7. Coury, C.: Hippocratic fingers and hypertrophic osteoarthropathy, *Brit J Dis Chest 54*:202-209, 1960.
8. Vogl, A., Blumenfeld, S., and Gutner, L. B.: Diagnostic significance of pulmonary hypertrophic osteoarthropathy, *Amer J Med 18*:51-65, 1955.
9. Vogl, A., and Goldfischer, S.: Primary or idiopathic osteoarthropathy, *Amer J Med 33*:166-187, 1962.
10. **Stone, O. J. Spoon nails and clubbing: significance mechanisms** *Cutis 16*:235-241, 1975.

CHAPTER 24

The Yellow Nail Syndrome

This nail dystrophy truly represents a manifestation of associated disease elsewhere. It was first brought to the awareness of clinicians by Samman and White[1] in 1964 as a marker for underlying respiratory and lymphoedema abnormalities.

It is characterized by:

1. Abnormal shape, color, nail plate quality and a decreased growth rate of the nail plate

2. Associated lymphoedema of lower extremities and either hereditary (Milroys) or acquired facial edema[2,3]

3. Upper and lower respiratory tract disease with or without plural effusion

4. Associated thyroid disease.

Table I summarizes the written literature on the association of other systems.

THE NAIL

Changes of the nail unit can occur at any age. There seems to be no sexual preference. It is remarkably more common and written about in England than in any other country. Only one patient reported is black.

Nail changes usually proceed pulmonary abnormalities, but nail changes caused by lymphoedema of lower extremities may exist for many years. These may spontaneously disappear, resulting in a normal nail unit (Fig. 7).

SHAPE

The nail plate in a full-blown case is usually hyperconvexed longitudinally as well as being laterally compressed (Figs. 1–3). Although the digit appears, at first glance, to be clubbed, there is a normal emergence angle and there is no softness of the proximal nail fold (Fig. 5). The latter may be edematous but lacks the pushability seen in clubbed fingers.

COLOR AND QUANTITY

A distinct yellow color can be appreciated but variations from lemon to dark yellow-green can be seen. Samman and White[5] have ruled out Pseudomonas as the contributor of the green color. The nail plate is opaque with the loss of its normal transparency (Figs. 1, 3, 6, 7). The nail plate is thickened (arrow-Fig. 3). The surface of the nail plate shows numerous tightly marked transversed ridges and shallow grooves (Figs. 1, 2). There is a reduced growth rate in these yellow nails. Samman and White[1] and Kandil[7] demonstrated this by different methods which measure nail plate growth. The nail plate may be onycholytic in its distal half (Figs. 4, 5); often, it is shed only to regrow yellow and thick again. The etiology of the thick, yellow slow-growing nail plate is unknown. Marks and Ellis[4] demonstrated that there was no statistically significant difference in the tissue clearing rates of proximal nail folds in normal patients and in patients with the yellow nail syndrome by using Iodinated (I^{131}) Serum Albumin. The literature is unconvincing that there are lymphatic abnormalities responsible for the nail unit abnormalities. Thyroid abnormalities have also been reported.

TREATMENT

Treatment appears to be unsatisfactory and spontaneous recovery rates of thirty percent have been described by Samman.[8] Intradermal injections (Dermo-Jet, 5 mg/cc Triamcinolone acetonide) in the proximal nail fold merit a trial according to Doctors Abell and Samman.[9] The use of Vitamin C has been reported helpful.[6]

Table I

Correlation of Other Systemic Signs In 73 Patients With Slow Growing, Thickened Yellow Nails: A Literature Review

	No. Patients	%
Edema lower extremities, includes Milroy's	56	76
Face Edema	34	46
Pleural Effusion	18	24
Chronic Bronchitis, Sinusitis, Bronchiectasis, and other upper and lower respiratory chronic disease	30	40
Only Yellow Nails	8	11

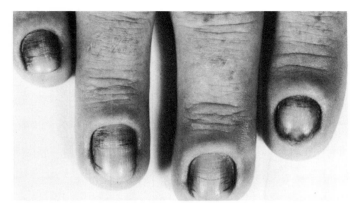

Fig. 1. Slow growing and opaque thickened fingers. Nails in 54-year-old Caucasian male with 6 months duration. No other systemic abnormalities present.

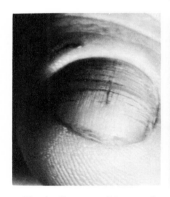

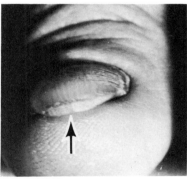

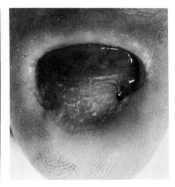

Fig. 2. Close up of fingernail showing characteristic grooving. This represents periods of nail growth which have been shown to be slower in this syndrome. U of M Derm.

Fig. 3. Thickened nail plate. U of M Derm.

Fig. 4. Thumb after avulsion of nail plate showing distal onycholysis. U of M Derm.

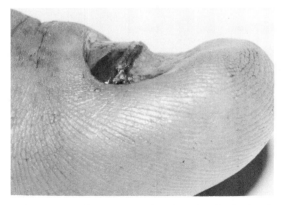

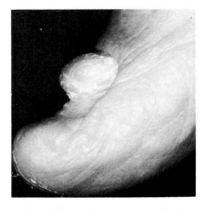

Fig. 5. Lateral view, same thumb as in Fig. 4, showing normal emergence angle of nail plate. U of M Derm.

Fig. 6. Very slow growing nail plate completely abnormal. Patient a 70-year-old Caucasian male. Asymptomatic 8 months duration.

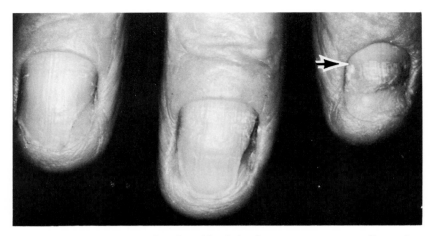

Fig. 7. Fingers of same patient from Fig. 6 showing spontaneous new nail growth. Asymptomatic.

NOTES

1 Saman, P.D. and White, W.F.: The yellow nail syndrome. *Brit. Jour. Derm.* 76: 153-157, 1964.

2. Emerson, P.A.: Yellow nails, lymphoedema and pleural effusions. *Thorax 21:* 247-253, 1966.

3. Dilley, J.J., Kierland, R.R., Randall, R.V. and Shick, R.M.: Primary lymphoedema associated with yellow nails and pleural effusions. *JAMA 204:* 122-125, 1968.

4. Marks, R. and Ellis, J.P.: Yellow nails. *Arch. Derm. 102:* 619-623, 1970.

5. Samman, P.D.: The yellow nail syndrome. *Tran. St. John Hosp. Derm. Soc. 59:* 37-38, 1973.

6. Ayres, S. and Mihan, R.: Yellow nail syndrome. *Arch. Derm. 108:* 267-268, 1973.

7. Kandil, E.: The yellow nail syndrome. *Jour. Int. Derm. 12:* 236-240, 1973.

8. Samman, P.D.: *The Nails in Disease,* 2nd Edition. Heinemann Medical Books, page 111.

9. Abell, E. and Samman, P.D.: Intradermal triancinolone acetonide injection in the yellow nail syndrome. *Transaction St. John Hosp. Derm. Soc. 59:* 114-117, 1973.

CHAPTER 25

Benign Tumors

FOCAL MYXOMATOUS DEGENERATION
(Synovial cyst, myxoid cyst)

These tumors are seen primarily in the distal phalanx where they may occur in the Proximal Nail Fold. Clinically, they are mostly asymptomatic, flesh-colored to red swellings (Fig. 1) which often have a translucent appearance (Fig. 2). Originally described[1] as synovial in origin, later investigators proved this not to be the case.[2-5] What appears to be a small cystic nodule will actually be serpentigenous and may extend for centimeters. When they occur over the nail matrix, they are space-occupying lesions and actually interfere with the production of nail plate from the most proximal matrix. The localized tumor causes the damaged nail plate to become a longitudinal groove (Fig. 2) or if it affects the matrix widely, they may form a series of transverse grooves (Fig. 3). The "tumor's" pressure damages the most proximal matrix reducing the matrix which results in a thinner nail plate. The tumor consists of a completely gelatinous transparent, glue-like material (Fig. 1).

TREATMENT

Patients who have pain, seek medical advice. All sorts of therapeutic regimens have been advocated: surgery, traumatizing it, and treating with all kinds of medications. By far the best of all of these, and yet inadequate, is the intralesional injection of corticosteroids. If one does not drain the material first it is not worth injecting. To drain the cyst, one needs a 16 gauge needle on a Luerlock tuberculin 1cc syringe. I've drained as much as 0.1 cc out. Draining is done from a proximal point (not a distal) of the tumor, otherwise on lowering the hands the opening where drained, will be inferior and all the steroid instilled injected will leak out.

I have used Triamcinolone Diacetate or Triamcinolone Acetonide-10,20 and 40 mg/cc. Often the intralesional injection has to be repeated four to five times. Injections are spaced over three week periods. Do not inject *deep* into the Proximal Nail Fold. I have seen localized atrophy after one injection (in Lichen Planus and myxomatous patients) (Figs. 4, 4a, 5).

SUBUNGUAL EXOSTOSIS AND INFLAMMATORY BONY PROLIFERATION

These tumors are uncommonly seen. They appear subungually on the great toes. They are slow to develop and are asymptomatic early (Figs. 6-12). A review of the last 30 years of the American Dermatologic literature[6-9] has collected thirteen patients. The evidence suggests that most lesions occur on the big toe (ten out of thirteen) following some sort of trauma.

Initially asymptomatic but later painful 13/13
History of no trauma preceding 3/13
Occuring through adolescence 8/13
More frequent in females 11/13

Diagnosis can be confirmed radiologically (Fig. 12). Histologic examination of a bony tumor reveals an inflamatory reaction surrounding the bone or the newly forming bone

Treatment—Conservative Treatment

Remove nail plate and curette the exostosis.

ENCHONDROMA

This rare tumor is composed of young cartilage, in the terminal phalanges.[10] When it starts subungually, it may deform the overlying nail plate. It has presented clinically as Paronychia.[11] It is slow growing and asymptomatic. Conservative treatment is indicated. Figures 13-15 present a patient who had a distal phalanx amputation.

FIBROMAS

Koenen's angio fibromas[12] are usually associated with tuberous sclerosis. These tumors may occur without evidence of tuberous sclerosis and perhaps may preceed other signs by many years.

These asymptomatic fibrous tumors may occur,[1] in the proximal nail fold near the matrix and spill over the matrix onto the nail plate, producing a longitudinal nail plate groove[2] in the matrix splitting the nail plate or[3] in the nail bed near the matrix, infiltrating and damaging the nail plate (Fig. 16).

The fibromas which are purely fibrous can be of two kinds:

1. *Fibrous digital tumors of children.*[13] Unusual fibromatous tumors originating at the terminal interphalangeal joint. These tumors present a Pseudosarcomatous histopathologic picture but they should be considered benign and conservatively removed.
2. *Garlic clove fibroma* is possibly the same as Koenen's. There are not enough reported cases to compare. Remove by conservative surgical techniques.

NEUROFIBROMA

Localized neurofibroma may occur in the Proximal Nail Fold producing a space-occupying lesion which will cause nail plate deformity, (Figs. 17-18). A single excision will suffice. Diffuse neurofibroma may enlarge the fingertip but cause minor nail unit abnormalities (Fig. 19).

VASCULAR TUMORS

Kaposi's hemorrhagic sarcoma may involve the nail bed by uplifting the nail plate and slightly deforming it.

GLOMUS TUMORS

Pain characterizes this uncommon nail bed tumor. Slow-growing glomus cells usually do not grow large but are extremely painful. Often not much is seen clinically in the nail bed; but with the right amount of lateral pressure to the distal phalanx, one can visualize a reddish macule, (Fig. 20). This small tumor is capable of bony erosion. (See Table I.) A diagnostic star-shaped telangectatic zone can be visualized by arteriography, but this is not routinely recommended.[15]

GRANULOMA TELANGECTATITUM (Pyogenic granuloma)

These fast growing vascular tumors can occur anywhere in the nail unit. Usually following a history of trauma, they may be painful and can destroy the bony phalanx.

If they originate in the Proximal Nail Fold matrix area, they will cause a localized nail plate defect (Figs. 21-22). In the nail bed, they will uplift the nail plate (Fig. 21). This tumor causes great patient anxiety since it's very painful and recurs.

Treatment should be conservative, destruction of a tumor either by cautery, freezing (liquid nitrogen) or Silver Nitrate (if no epidermis is present).

EPIDERMAL BUDS

These tumors usually are miscroscopic in size and rarely produce symptoms. Samman[16] was the first to describe them. Lewin[17] affirms that they may occur more frequently than we think. One patient did grow a large one destroying the nail plate and upsetting the nail bed. A warty growth thought to be a malignant melanoma was in fact an epidermoid bud. These may also occur in clubbed fingers.[17]

EPIDERMAL CYSTS OF NAIL BED (Epidermoid cyst of phalanx)

These tumors are rarely seen by dermatologists. They arise in the tip of the terminal phalanx invariably at the site of past trauma. A disfiguring growth remains asymptomatic until the expanding cyst pressures the phalanx bony plate and causes its fracture. Pain now becomes a major concern to the patient. Bone lytic lesions are seen.

Hystologically, the tumor has a typical epidermal cyst architecture. Single excision or curettage will suffice.

Verrucous Epidermal Hyperplasia

Verrucous epidermal hyperplasia may react as a space-occupying lesion and destroy the phalanx; and if it occurs on the nail bed, uplift the nail plate. This condition has been described by Hartman[18] in a patient who had Incontinentia pigmenti when younger. The tumor was characterized by Pseudo-Epitheliomatous hyperplasia, hyperkeratosis, hypergranulosis, some parakeratosis and "Dyskeratosis."

Under the name of Distinctive, Destructive Digital Disease, A.A. Fisher[19] has described and followed one patient who appears to have a similar subungal process. Dr. Fisher's case apparently showed more parakeratosis. This could represent a Keratoacanthoma.

Probably the patient described by Shapiro and Stoller[20] as having subungual wart with phalanx erosion also suffered this entity. The authors describe a dyskeratosis in lower epidermis with a warty surface. This could represent a Keratoacanthoma. These lesions are painful, and may occur from one finger to another. Clinically, they appear as subungual warts.

VERRUCA VULGARIS

Warts on the nail unit perimeter are by no means "Vulgaris." As a characteristic, they resist treatment, tormenting patient and doctor alike.

Verrucas arise in epidermis that has a granular layer. As exceptions, the verruca-like lesion of the oral aspects of the lips are noted. These as yet have not been reconfirmed to be due to Popova virus.

In any event, periungual warts may ring the entire nail field area, (Fig. 25). With time, the nail bed may be invaded for a short distance. Verruca commonly involve the PNF and may also occur in the ventral epidermal surface of the proximal nail fold, (Figs. 26-28).

Warts may grow very large, eroding the bony phalanx (See Table I).[21,22] Treatment is difficult. Cures have been claimed by; (1) use of Methotrexate in large doses,[23] (2) DNCB sensitization, (3) hypnosis with curative results, (4) Bleomycin intralesionally[24] and (5) Liquid Nitrogen or other destructive measures (Fig. 29).

Avulsion of the nail plate is favored, as better destruction of the periungual tissues are achieved.

The reported cases[24] of warts occurring in immune defect states are most likely true but probably secondary to systemic Prednisone given for treatment of the immune disease. Another example is patients taking Prednisone for Fogo Salvagem, (Pemphigus Erythematosus) who develop a higher incidence of widespread verrucas.

CUTANEOUS HORN

Very rare pigmented cutaneous horn arising from matrix-nail bed is in Fig. 30. Removal after avulsion was curative.

Table I

Tumors capable of phalanx erosion

Warts—Epidermal
Verrucous epidermal hyperplasia
Glomus
Exostosis
Enchondroma
Granuloma telangectaticum
Keratoacanthoma
Squamous cell carcinoma

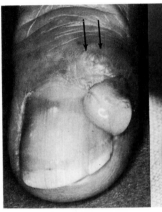
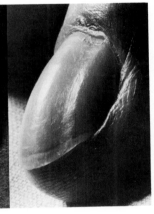
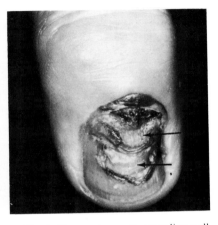

Fig. 1. Focal myxomatous degeneration. Space in proximal nail fold must be evacuated of this gel-like material usually 15-16 gauge needle and 1 cc. tuberculin syringe prior to infiltration with steroids.

Fig. 2. Focal myxomatous degeneration. A space occupying lesion has pressured the matrix focally and produced a longitudinal grooved nail plate.

Fig. 3. Myxomatous cyst, extending well into the PNF and close to the joint (see arrows) produced dystrophy of nail plate in a swirl pattern.

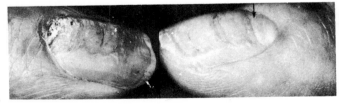
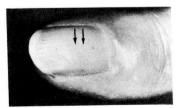

Fig. 4. Myxomatous cyst, dammaging nail plate.

Fig. 4a Lesion of Fig. 4 after 2 months. 0.05 cc 20mg/cc steroid 1.L. PNF.

Fig. 5. Same as in Figure 4, three months after I.L. injection of Triamcinolone acetonide 20 mg/cc. Note small area of atrophy (double arrow) remnants of dystrophic nail plate is seen distal to arrow.

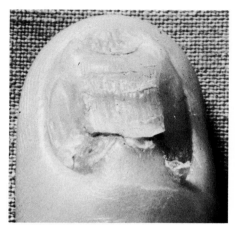

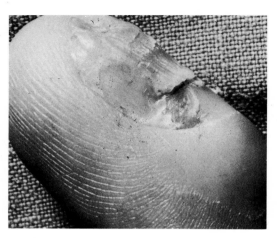

Fig. 6. **Subungual exostosis following frac-**ture of distal phalanx. University of Miami, Dept. of Dermatology.

Fig. 7. Side view of finger in Fig. 6. PNF feels boney hard. Dermatology Department, University of Miami.

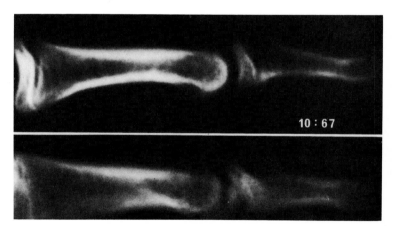

Fig. 8. X-rays of phalanx on 10:67. Note fracture and exostosis on 1:68. Department of Dermatology, University of Miami.

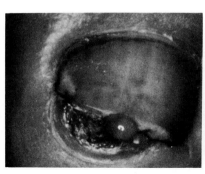

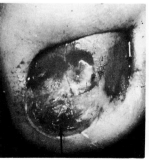

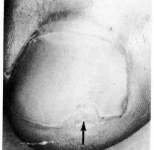

Fig. 9. Clinical presentation subungual exostosis. Painful exudative subungual process which is chronic in nature, 12 year old male.

Figure 10. Same patient as in figure 9 with nail off. Biopsy from area of arrow.

Fig. 11. **Earliest clinical pre-**sentation. Subungual exostosis, arrow.

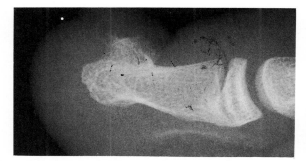

Fig. 12. X-ray of subungual exostasis.

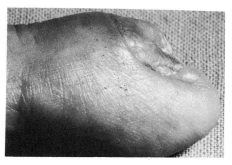

Fig. 13. Clinical presentation of Enchondroma. Very slow growing asymptomatic.

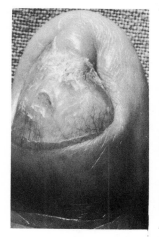

Fig. 14. Same patient as in Fig. 13.

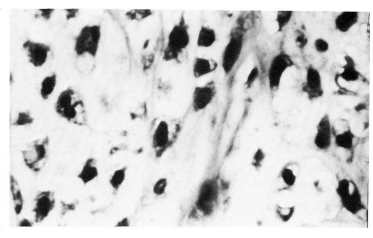

Fig. 15. Photomicrograph enchondroma, showing mature cartilage cells. H&E X1600.

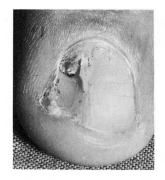

Fig. 16. Intraungual Fibroma.

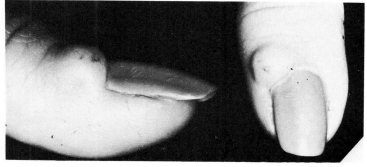

Fig. 17. Neurofibroma of PNF. Note longitudinal grooving of nail plate. (Courtesy Dr. P. Frost)

Fig. 18. Neurofibroma. Same patient as in Figure 17. (Courtesy Dr. P. Frost)

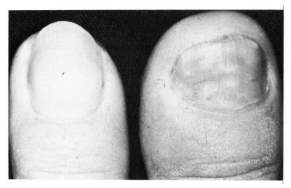

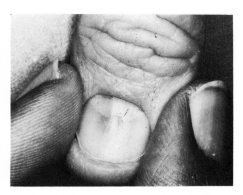

Fig. 19. Generalized neurofibroma of thumb. Compare with normal opposite thumb, same patient.

Fig. 20. Glomus tumor, symptomatic sharp pain on trauma. Red area of nail bed only when there is lateral pressure as shown.

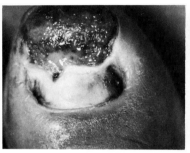

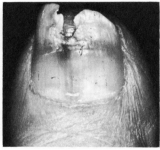

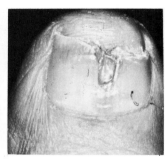

Fig. 21. Pyogenic granuloma, distally. uplifted nail plate. University of Miami, Department of Dermatology.

Fig. 22. Clinical appearance of pyogenic granuloma. Very painful. Note mid nail plate erosion distally and opaque lytic area proximally.

Fig. 23. Same patient as in Figure 25. All areas that appeared lytic were removed.

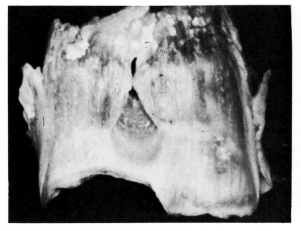

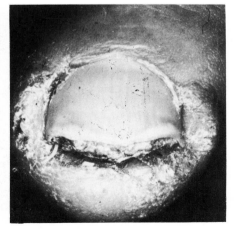

Fig. 24. Nail plate underside. Note origin of Pyogenic granuloma at matrix-nail bed border. In retrospect it must have been much larger earlier and resulted in the erosion at the distal nail plate.

Fig. 25. Warts in lateral nail fold with nail bed involvement.

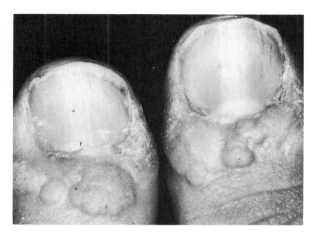

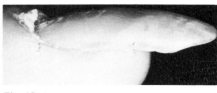

Fig. 27. PNF wart, side view.

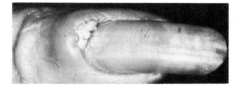

Fig. 26. PNF warts.

Fig. 28. PNF wart.

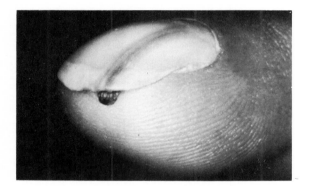

Fig. 29. Periungual wart treated with liquid nitrogen. Hemorrhage often may occur.

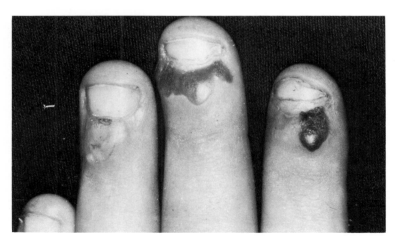

Fig. 30. Nail bed cutaneous horn, pigmented. Single excision at lunula was curative, histologically it was a papilloma.

NOTES

1. Mackee, T. and Andrew, G.: Synovial Lesion of the skin. *Arch Derm & Syph* 4:162, 1921.
2. Montgomery, R. and Culver, R.: Synovial Cysts of the fingers. *Arch Derm Syph 5*: 329, 1922.
3. **Woodburne, A.R.: The Yellow-Nail Syndrome *Arch Derm Symp* 407, 1947.**
4. Smith, E.B., Skipworth, G.B., Vander Poleg, D.E.: Longitudinal grooving of nails due to synovial cysts. *Arch Derm* 89: 364-366, 1964.
5. Roth, W.G., Obrenovic, A., Weber, G.: Quistes Synoviales Subungueales *Dermatologia Revista Mexicana* 12: 5-10, 1968.
6. Cortijo, A.T., Pons, S., Bellene, R.N.: Manifest-aciones cutaneous de las exostosis. *Dermatologia Iben Latino Americana*. 11: 41-48, 1969.
7. Cohen, H.J., Frank, S.B., Minikin, W., Gibbs, R.C.: Subungual exostosis. *Arch Derm* 107: 431-432, 1973.
8. Lebovitz, S.S., Miller, O.F., Dickey, R.F.: Subungual exostosis *Cutis* 13: 426-428, 1974.
9. **Zimmerman, E.H. Subungual Exostosis *Cutis* 19: 185-188, 1977.**
10. Yaffee, H.S.: Peculiar nail dystrophy caused by an Enchondroma. *Arch Derm* 91: 361, 1965.
11. Shelley, W.B., Ralston, E.L.: Paronychia due to an Endchondroma. *Arch Derm* 90: 412-413, 1964.
12. Steel, H.H.: Garlic clove fibroma *J.A.M.A.* 191: 1082-1083, 1965.
13. **Reye, R.D.K.: Recurring digital fibrous tumors of childhood. *Arch Path* 80: 228-231, 1965.**
14. Masson, P.: Le glomus neuromyo-arterial des regions tactiles et ses tumeurs. *Lyons CHR* 21: 257-280, 1924.
15. Camirand, P., Giroux, J.M.: Subungual glomus tumor *Arch Derm* 102: 677-679, 1970.
16. **Samman, P.D.: The human toenail; its genesis and blood supply. *Br. J. Derm.* 71: 296-302, 1952.**
17. **Lewin, K.: Subungual epidermoid inclusions. *Br. J. Derm.* 81: 671-675, 1969.**
18. **Hartman, D.L.: Incontinentia pigment associated with subungual tumors. *Arch Derm* 94: 632-635, 1966.**
19. Fisher, A.A.: A distinctive, destructive digital disease, *Arch Derm* 83: 1030-1031, 1961.
20. **Shapiro, A. and Stoller, R.: Erosion of phalanges by subgungual warts. *J.A.M.A.* 176: 379, 1961.**
21. Plegwig, G., Christophers, E., Braun-Falco, O: Mutilating subungual warts. *Hautarzt* 24: 338-341, 1973.
22. Gardner, L.W., Acker, D.W.: Bone destruction of a distal phalanx caused by periungual warts. *Arch Derm* 107: 275-276, 1973.
23. Perry, T.L., Harman, L.J.: Warts in diseases with immune defect. *Cutis* 13: 359-362, 1974.
24. **Bremmer, R.M.: Warts: treatment with intralesional bleonycin. *Cutis* 18: 264-266, 1976.**
25. Rees, T.D. and Trier, W.C. Epithelial inclusion cysts of thumb phalanx. *British J. Plast Surg.* 12: 323-326, 1960.

CHAPTER 26

Malignant Tumors

PREMALIGNANT LESIONS

Arsenical Keratosis

Clinically, a Keratotic papule or plaque on the lateral nail fold or nail bed, could appear unaccompanied by a history of either iatrogenic arsenic ingestion. Histopathologically, it is similar to that seen in skin lesions, particularly the termed hyperplastic actinic Keratosis.

In patients with iatrogenic arsenic intake or in patients inhabiting a geographic area high in environmental arsenic (certain zones in Argentina, Taiwan and Europe), other signs of arsenicalism may also occur.

The nail unit, however, presents with Keratotic papules and plaques which are subungual causing dystrophy to the overlying nail plate.

KERATOSIS RESULTING FROM PAST USE OF IONIZING RADIATION

This lesion is commonly seen in patients who were treated with x-rays for Onychomycosis and hand eczemas twenty to thirty-five years prior to showing signs (Figs. 1-4). Also, physicians who used fluroscopic techniques may develop a variety of lesions ranging from benign Keratosis of the palm skin (Fig. 5.) to frank Squamous Cell Carcinoma of the nail bed area.

The earliest premalignant lesions noted in the nail bed are red longitudinal striations starting at the lunula resulting in minimal longitudinal nail plate ridges (Figs. 1-4).

Keratotic papules develop at the border of the lateral nail fold and the nail bed. These lesions extend to the lanula and eventually destroy the matrix resulting in no nail plate. Although the lesions may originate in the lunula, the nail bed becomes Keratotic and Verrucous.

A slow progression (years) is usually the course. Pain occurs late in the disease (Figs. 3, 4).

Histopathology varies from the papilloma with unusual atypia of nuclei in the Basal Cell layer to a great deal of dyskeratosis throughout.

Treatment should be very conservative. Usually destruction of lesions leaving adequate borders suffices to produce a cure. Personally, I have found freezing to be an excellent treatment modality.

MALIGNANT TUMORS

See Table I (Radial growth of squamous cell in nail bed).

INTRAEPIDERMAL CELL CARCINOMA (BOWEN'S DISEASE)

This premalignant lesion is not as rare as the medical literature makes it appear. I, personally, have treated ten cases. It is probable that a nail bed Squamous Cell Carcinoma will always start as intraepithelial Squamous Cell Carcinoma. Both of these diseases have a slow progressive course; and patients with intraepidermal Squamous Cell Carcinoma have shown invasion and a frank change, to Squamous Cell Carcinoma. The lesions may start anywhere in the nail bed (Fig. 6) or lunula junction and extend peripherally. The invasion of the proximal nail fold with the formation of "a whitish band" is characteristic (Fig. 7 arrows).

This only represents the involved dyskeratotic skin of the proximal nail fold. The clinician should immediately think of intraepidermal cell carcinoma on seeing the nail plate sharply demarcated with nail bed hyperplasia and proximal nail fold epidermal abnormalities (Figs. 6,7).

A biopsy should be done in the most indurated and verrucous area and not in the easy to biopsy borders, as you will miss an already invasive Squamous Cell Carcinoma.[1]

Treatment of choice is Moh's chemosurgery or dermatologic conventional desiccation and curettage. Always avulse the nail plate for easier access. Amputation and grafts are unnecessary. 5-flurouracil produces great morbidity. X-ray treatment makes no sense.

BASAL CELL CARCINOMA[2]

Probably the rarest of epidermal tumors affecting the nail matrix and nail bed behaves like a basal cell elsewhere. Treatment should be conservative, amputation is not necessary. Moh's chemosurgery is the treatment of choice.

SQUAMOUS CELL CARCINOMA

This is perhaps the most common of all nail unit tumors except malignant melanoma. This tumor also exhibits radial and vertical growth phases. The radial phase may be long lasting—10 to 15 years.

It is a slow growing tumor which probably originates in the nail bed and invades the matrix and lateral nail fold (Fig. 8). A patient's history characteristically is of years of treatment for an "infection" (Fig. 9) or a "Paronychia." Matrix and/or paronychial involvement may result in painful episodes. Redness and paronychial swelling are confused with infections (Fig. 9), There are two special situations of which the clinician should be aware:

1) A history of ionizing radiation to the hands of the patient; and potential tumor.

2) congenital epidermal dysplasia.

Both of these result in a graver prognosis from an otherwise biologically low-malignant potentially tumor.

Usually benign-squamous cell carcinoma occurs in patients 50-75 years of age. In patients with epidermal dysplasia, however, earlier appearances of nail unit squamous cell carcinoma occur with a more malignant disposition. Metastasis of that can be terminal for the patient[3,4]

Also, patients who received x-ray therapy for hand eczema or Onychomycosis years earlier and physicians who used fluroscopic equipment are predisposed to develop squamous cell carcinoma of the digits and hands (Figs. 10,11).

Although there is no large study written anywhere in the medical literature, it is believed that squamous cell carcinoma secondary to ionizing radiation may matastasize earlier than that of a patient who has absolutely no predisposing past history.

The clinician should suspect tumor whenever a nail unit lesion which is destructive does not heal in a period of not more than 3-6 months (Figs. 9-12).

Squamous cell carcinoma can also develop in Bowen's lesions as stated previously. Histologically, it is a low grade type malignancy (Figs. 13, 14, 15).

The biologic concept of squamous cell carcinoma of the nail bed beginning as an intraepithelial carcinoma (radial growth phase) and becoming invasive later (vertical growth rate) can be theorized.

Table I
Summarizes Signs and Symptoms of all Malignant Tumors.

INTRAEPITHELIAL LESIONS
  1) Arsenical Keratosis
  2) Keratosis Secondary to Radiotherapy
  3) Intraepithelial Squamous Cell Carcinoma (Bowen's Disease)

MALIGNANT TUMORS
LOCALIZED
  1) Basal Cell Carcinoma
  2) Keratoacanthoma
    a) Solitary
    b) Ferguson-Smith
  3) Squamous Cell Carcinoma
    a) Idiopathic
    b) Hereditary Ectodermal Dysplasia
    c) After Radiotherapy
  4) Metastatic Lesion
    Lung, Breast, Colon, Kidney
  5) Malignant Melanoma
  6) Mycosis Fungoides
  7) Histiocytosis—X

Invasion of the underlying phalanx with destruction is not common but it occurs.

TREATMENT

Local destruction by electrodesiccation and curettage, or Moh's chemosurgery is indicated. Amputation, as a last resort, should be done in carefully selected cases.

KERATOACANTHOMA (KA)

Nail unit Keratoacanthoma is most commonly confused as a squamous cell carcinoma. The features of a KA are distinctly and characteristically different from squamous cell carcinoma.

Two types of KA occur:

1) The appearance of a KA tumor in the nail unit in a patient who has multiple disseminated KA of the Ferguson-Smith type (Fig. 16);

2) A solitary KA of the nail unit. (This lesion is usually confused for a squamous cell carcinoma). Clinically, it is symptomatic (painful) in weeks rather than years of onset. It produces a red swelling of the tip of the terminal phalanx and results usually in a destructive bone lesion.[5]

Maculay[6] has reviewed the subject well and has incorporated such clinical entities as Fisher's "Distinctive, Destructive Digital Disease" as Keratoacanthomata.

Treatment may present a problem because of the extent of the tumor on the digit tip. Local destruction may not be complete and the tumor may recur. Lyctic bone lesions heal themselves; cryotherapy may be used. Amputation should be a last resort.

Table II summarizes duration signs and symptoms of lesions.

METASTATIC DISEASE TO THE NAIL AND FINGER TIP

Metastasis to the nail unit or tip of digit by other neoplasm is rare. More often than not these phalangeal metastases are the initial symptoms of an otherwise silent malignancy.

The most common metastases are from lung, breast and colon.

An updated computation of reported metastasis follows:

Lung	20	- (7,8)
Breast	5	- (9)
Colon	4	- (7,10)
Kidney	2	

One case each of parotid, testis, plasma cell myeloma, skin, adrenal, neuroblastoma and undertermined metastasis.

MELANOCYTIC LESIONS

Malignant melanoma of the subungual area is without a doubt a very serious and life threatening disease. It, however, carries a much better prognosis when compared to malignant melanoma of other skin areas. The biologic concepts surrounding the diagnosis of melanocyte lesions termed melanoma are gradually being clarified, these are summarized elsewhere.

PIGMENTED MELANOCYTIC LESIONS

For an expanded discussion of pigmented lesions of melanocytic origin, see addenda at the end of this chapter.

Incidence, Race, Sex

The Temple University Melanoma Study Group[1] reports that approximately 5.6 per cent of cutaneous melanomas studied occur in the volar and subungual site! Other reported incidences vary from 5—10 percent.[2-4] The incidence of all cutaneous melanomas in blacks is very low and is summarized by Elwood and Lee[5] to be about 1 percent. The curious fact about it is that malignant melanomas occuring in the soles and subungual area are seen in 25 percent of blacks.[6] As Clark has stated, "Malignant melanomas in blacks occur mostly below the ankles or on the oral mucous membrane." Later in this chapter we will talk about acral lentiginous melanoma. Are Blacks more susceptible to this biologic type of melanoma?

The clinical appearance and the prognosis of pigmented lesions of the subungual area can be separated into at least four types:

1. Normal pigmented nail plate bands in Caucasians and Orientals (PNB) (Figs. 17-21)
2. Acral lentiginous melanomas (ALM)[7]
3. Superficial spreading melanomas (SSMM) (very rare on subungual?)[1](Figs. 22-25)
4. Nodular melanomas (NM) (Fig. 26)
5. Congenital and rare syndromes of childhood melanoma (very rare)

Pigmented Nail plate Bands (PNB) Benign

Not enough data is available today to clearly relate all pigmented nail plate bands in non-blacks to malignant melanoma. Pigmented bands start commonly in children and younger adults. Melanoma is uncommonly seen in this age group but it occurs commonly in the 40 and over age group.

Clinically PNB start as a beige to brown longitudinal band of the nail plate, (Fig. 17, Chart B,BB). As time goes on the width of this band widens and often the color increases in intensity becoming darker brown, (Fig. 20, Chart C, CC, D, DD) and after many years black, (Figs. D, DD). What produces the pigmented band in children? My own experience and that of others is that a nidus of "melanocytes" in the matrix incorporates melanin granules into the corresponding nail plate site. They may increase in numbers and the pigmented granules are markedly increased along the long dendrites of the cells—let's say "melanocytic hyperplasia." No abnormal cytologic details are noted, (Figs. 20, 21). Can these lentiginous aggregates form "theques"? Can they be called junction nevus?

Very little published data can be relied on which specifically answers these questions. In my own series of 6 biopsies (3 children and 3 adults) no theques were seen but rather "lentiginous" melanocytes.

In summary, pigmented bands are seen in younger rather than older individuals. Their color is uniform and reduced in intensity—one can almost see through them. They may be light beige or light brown; these do not become malignant melanoma in younger patients. But will they become melanomas later in life? Again, very little is written about this: I would be concerned if a pigmented band occured first at a later age group (40 and over). Recent widening of the biologic concepts of melanomas specifically those which have first a radial growth phase for years, (i.e. acral lentiginous melanoma, superficial spreading melanoma and lentigo maligina melanoma) and then a vertical phase growth—which is prognostically worse, have allowed the physician to prognosticate and treat more realistically. One can only wonder and strongly suspect that the widening pigmented nail plate band is, in fact, the radial growth of one of these special melanomas. This may be circumstantially supported by the high incidence of malignant melanoma in the same patients. And furthermore, the higher incidence of melanoma in older patients who may or may not have had a previous pigmented band since childhood.

Should one take these pigmented bands out as soon as one diagnoses them? The answer to this question in my opinion is "yes." It needs only one qualification and that is to be sure it is widening. Care must be shown not to create a greater problem to the patient than what he has. No radical or extended excisions are needed. This lesion is *intraepidermal* and conventional methods may be used for example (1) avulsion of the nail plate and destruction of the epidermis either by cautery or similar methods or even freezing, (2) excession of focus in matrix can also be done. From the therapeutic view the sooner this is done, the smaller the scar will be.

Acral Lintiginous Melanoma (ALM)

What is an acral lentiginous melanocytic lesion? Statistical data as well as histologic data have presented what seems to be a unique biologic type of melanocytic lesion. The occurrence in the volar-plantar areas where the epidermis is again different than that of the skin elsewhere possibly suggests a different melanocytic, as well as keratinocytic, cell for that skin. It is interesting to note that squamous cell carcinoma of the subungual area behaves as if there were an initial radial growth phase which is intraepidermal exclusively (Bowen's) and after many years (10-15) invasion or vertical growth phase is noted. This fact has been described[8] and I have noted two cases of my own.

Histologically, in melanocytic lesions (ALM and SSMM) The difference lies in the behavior of the "active" melanocyte. In ALM the activity first is basilar as compared with SSMM where the activity starts in the basal cell layer but quickly involves the entire thickness of the epidermis[1] (see Table I.)

Nail Plate Color Changes from Light to Darker

1. This clinical picture already implies alteration of the matrix epidermis and represents more advanced stages. If the patient relates a history of having a pigmented band uniformally pigmented for many years and now a change has occured, very likely it represents a more advanced stage of either Acral lentiginous melanoma or the rarer is subungual superficial spreading malignant melanoma. Very scanty data exists to differentiate these two conditions in the matrix. The anatomic (physical) structure of the nail matrix and its nail plate in fact, interfere (Figs. A, AA, B, BB, C, CC, D, DD).

2. The nail plate will reflect early papular or nodular aggregation of melanocytic pigmented cells in the matrix as streaks of darker pigmented color will be apparent in the nail plate (Figs. E, EE).

Regardless, these lesions are not commonly seen in younger patients. Radial growth phase of matrix lesions not only produces wider bands but also involvement of the proximal nail fold epithelium with the resultant sign—Hutchison's sign.

Hutchison's sign consists of the leaching of melanin pigment into the PNF. It may also be seen in nodular melanomas and should not be considered a benign sign (Figs. F, FF).

3. Nail Plate changes such as destruction of the plate are graver signs and command swift action. More advanced radially growing melanomas, (Figs. 21, F, FF, G, GG) (now nodular?) or those melanomas quickly becoming nodular from their inception produce nail plate changes.

4. Melanomas which are as prominant in the nail bed as they are in the matrix probably represent lesions which are not the delayed forming types (ALM or SSMM) but rather nodular. They are historically of short durations, 6 months to 1 year and are very destructive.

Amelanotic malignant melanomas are of this type and are usually confused by the clinician as fungus or other benign problems (Fig. 25).

Melanomas rapidly aggressive of childhood remain a rarity. Table II summarizes signs, symptoms and histologic appearance of most pigmented nail neoplasms.

Prognosis and Treatment

The reader should refer to Clark et. al.[1] for more details; but, generally:

1. Tumors with only radial growth have a better prognosis than those with an added vertical growth.

2. Tumors with only a radial growth are given a Level II grade and are measured (thickness). If this thickness is less than 0.76 mm the prognosis is excellent if excised.

3. Tumors with only radial growth phase that are 0.76 mm to 1.5 mm, to the best educated guess, have to recur 10 to 30 % after excision.

4. Tumors with both a radial and vertical growth phase or only a vertical growth phase greater than 1.5 mm have a graver prognosis, 50% recurrence. Although data is still being gathered, Clark and associates believe that there should be a regional lymph node dissection.

Table II
Duration, Signs, and Symptoms of Common Pre-Malignant and Malignant Nail Lesions

Description	Duration	Pain	Remarks	Treatment
Actinic, Arsenical or Radiation Keratosis	Many years	Very late	Predisposing history	Epidermal destruction only—freezing
Intra-epithelial Squamous Cell Carcinoma	Many years	Late	Usually no history of predisposing factors	Epidermal destruction—freezing or curetting
Squamous Cell Carcinoma	Many Years	Late	55-70 age group May or may not have predisposing factors (Bone destruction by invasion)	Amputation rarely needed—local destruction or surgical or chemosurgical procedures
Keratoacanthoma	Weeks	Early	Usually 30-50 year age group (Bone destruction by pressure)	Conservative—freezing
Basal Cell	Many years	Late	Rarest	Conservative

Table III

Comparative Histologic Features of the Radial Growth Phases of Acral Lentiginous, Superficial Spreading and Lentigo Maligna Types

	Acral Lentiginous Melanoma	Lentigo Maligna Melanoma	Superficial Spreading Melanoma
Location of Melanoma Cells within the Epidermis	Basilar region	Basilar region	All epidermal layer
Cytology of the Individually Disposed Intra-Epidermal Melanocytes	Uniformly large with prominant, complex dendrites	Pleomorphic- "Normal" and bizarre melanocytes mixed. Dendrites inconspicuous	Uniformly large epithelioid cells without prominent dendrites
History of the Intra-epidermal Nests of Melanocytes	Nests tend to bulge into dermis	Nests may be ellipsoidal in outline with the long axis tending to parallel the epidermal surface	Nests quite large frequently bridging the entire thickness of the epidermis
Cytology of the Melanocytes forming the Intra epidermal Nests	Cells tend to be spindle-shaped, may be epithelioid	Cells are pleomorphic; some quite small, others large and bizarre	Uniformly large epithelioid cells from the nests.
Invasion of the Papillary Dermis	Present, but may require search to find it	Essentially absent	Easily demonstrated
Solar Changes in Connective Tissue	Absent	Present	Variable
Host Response of Lymphocytes and Macrophages	Present and prominent with extension into epidermis	Minimal to absent	Usually well developed

From: Clark, Bernardino, Reed and Kopf 1978[1]

When Should Regional Node Dissection Be Done?

Clark and associates[1] recommend regional node dissections be done in:
1. "Stage II disease (clinical);" 2. "Level IV and V disease regardless of thickness;" and 3. "All tumors with a thickness greater than 1.50 mm."

SYSTEMIC NEOPLASMS

Mycosis Fungoides

This systemic "T" cell neoplasm can produce nail plate shedding and nail bed hypertrophy (figs. 27, 28). Histopathology of the nail lesion is identical to that of skin.

Histocytosis—X

This systemic Histocytosis usually involves the scalp, (Fig. 29) and frequently may involve the Proximal nail fold, matrix and nail bed. The lesions look typically like those of Lichen Planus including Vickham's striae (Fig. 21) and nail plate atrophy (Fig. 30, 31).

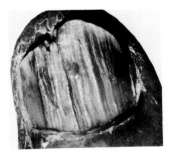

Fig. 1. Post radiation matrix, minimal damage with nail plate ridging.

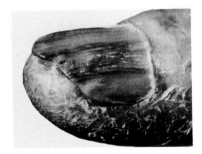

Fig. 2. Lateral view of same finger as in Figure 1.

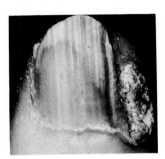

Fig. 3. Keratotic lesion subungual starting at lateral margin of nail bed. Post radiation damage.

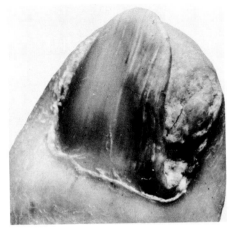

Fig. 4. Same lesion in fig 3 - 5 years later. Histopathology resembles Actinic Keratosis.

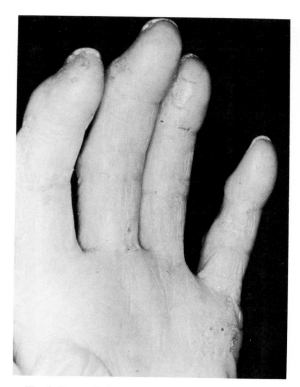

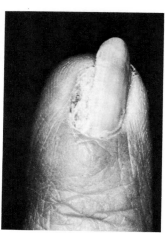

Fig. 6. Intra-epidermal Squamous Cell Carcinoma involving nail bed, matrix, (no nail plate), and PNF of one half of finger only. Sharp delineation of matrix is clue to tumor.

Fig. 5. Post radiation Keratosis, hand.

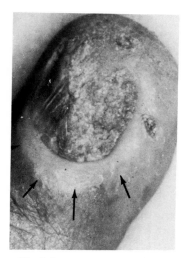

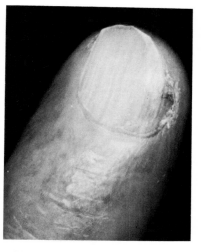

Fig. 7. Intra-epidermal Squamous Cell Carcinoma, more estensive lesion involving nail bed, matrix and proximal nail fold (white band sign), arrows, serial sectioning of lesion may often show early invasive squamous cell carcinoma.

Fig. 8. Squamous cell carcinoma, short duration, location easily confuses physician to think fungus rather than tumor. Lesions longer than 3 - 6 months should be biopsied.

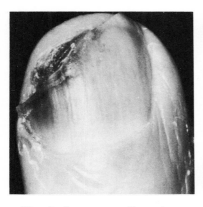

Fig. 9. Squamous cell carcinoma. Four years duration. Occasionally even Candida albicans and as in this case Pseudomonas will colonize subungual niche.

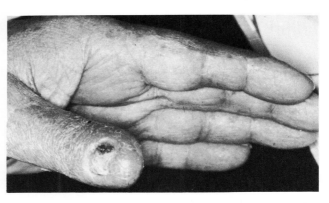

Fig. 10. Squamous cell carcinoma on thumb nail of physician who used fluroscopic techniques in past.

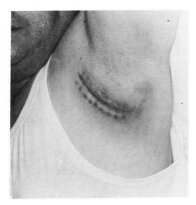

Fig. 11. **Metastatic lymph node,** same patient as Figure 10. Keratotic hands ten years prior to Metastosis. Well differentiated squamous cell carcinoma.

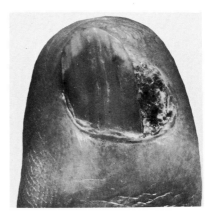

Fig. 12. **Squamous cell carcinoma.** 5 year duration. Clue to tumor etiology is sharp marginations of matrix destruction (nail plate), absent nail plate in lesion.

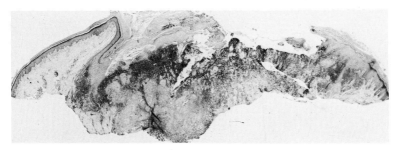

Fig. 13. **Photomicrograph of longitudinal biopsy of lesion, Figure 12, extending** from PNF to hyponychium. H&E X16.

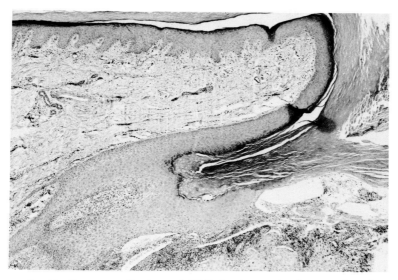

Fig. 14. Closer magnifications of PNF showing no involvement there but squamous cell tumor destroying matrix, arrow. H&E X220.

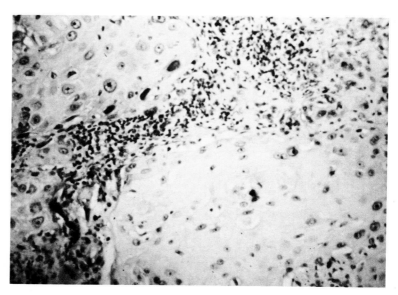

Fig. 15. Higher magnification of invasive cords of squamous cell carcinoma. H&E X800.

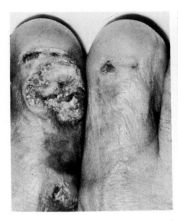

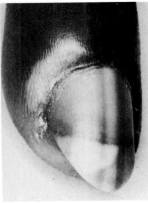

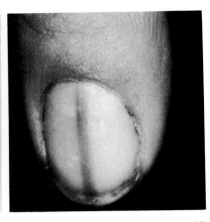

Fig. 16. Fergusson-Smith keratoacanthoma involving great toe on left and previously right toe with great destruction. Keratoacanthomas single or multiple are very destructive of bone and structures they overlie. (Courtesy of Dr. Fabio Londono.)

Fig. 17. Pigmented band in black female. Very common.

Fig. 18. Pigmented band in 12 year old boy. Very rare.

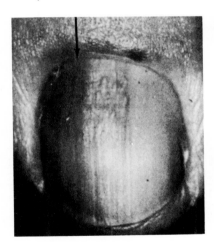

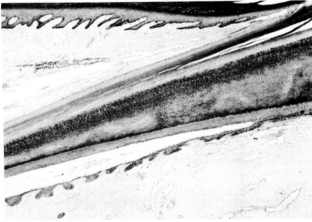

Fig. 19. Very wide pigmented band in Caucasin male who also had Addison's Disease. Band widened to size shown in figure in past four years.

Fig. 20. Photomicrograph of biopsy taken from finger in Figure 18, showing proximal nail fold (PNF), nail plate (NP) and matrix (M). X120 Silver H&E

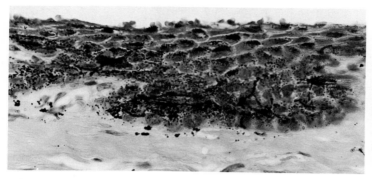

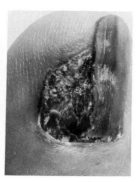

Fig. 21. Photomicrograph at higher magnification of arrow in Figure 18 showing abundant normal appearing melanocytes in matrix. Silver X 800.

Fig. 22. Malignant melanoma. 18 month duration.

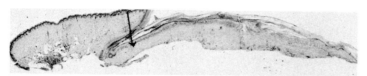

Fig. 23. Photomicrograph of longitudinal biopsy of Figure 22, (arrow) showing melanoma involving nail bed, matrix but not proximal nail fold (PNF). H&E X16.

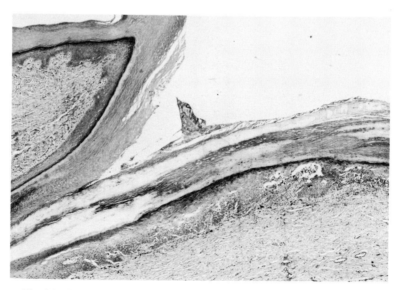

Fig. 24. Photomicrograph of biopsy in Figure 22 showing epidermal involvement of matrix and nail bed with atypical and malignant melanocytes. H&E X240.

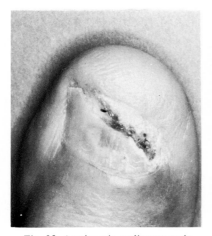

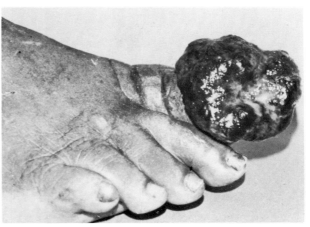

Fig. 25. Amelanotic malignant melanoma. 14 month duration. Misdiagnosed as mycosis. Physician should note a change in 2-3 months maximum if culture is positive. Amputation, five year survival.

Fig. 26. Malignant melanoma, three years duration. Regional nodes involved. (Courtesy of Dr. F. Battistini.)

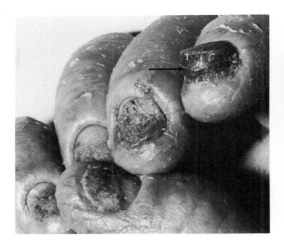

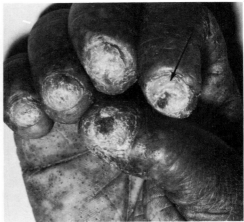

Fig. 27. Mycosis fungoides. Terminal stages. Marked nail bed hyperplasia with most nail plates off but one, arrow.

Fig. 28. Mycosis fungoides. Regrowth of nail plate is possible, arrow.

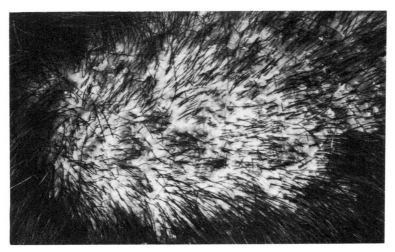

Fig. 29. Histiocytosis-X, 14-year-old male with scalp involvement; patient referred by Dr. Victor Torres.

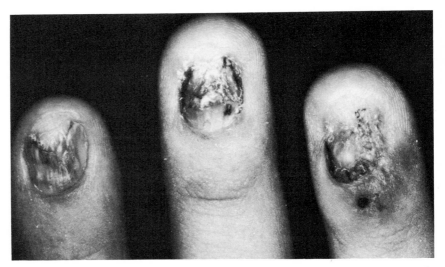

Fig. 30. Histiocytosis-X fingers of same patient as in figure 30 showing proximal nail fold (arrow) and matrix resulting in nail plate atrophy. Histology proven patient referred Dr. Victor Torres.

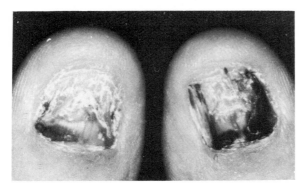

Fig. 31. Histiocytosis-X; thumbs of same patient.

ADDENDUM

PIGMENTED LESIONS OF MELANOCYTIC ORIGIN

Malignant melanoma of the subungual area is without a doubt a very serious and life threatening disease. However, it carries a much better prognosis when compared to malignant melanoma of other skin areas. The biologic concepts surrounding the diagnosis of melanocyte lesions termed melanoma are gradually being clarified. These are summarized further on.

Caucasians normally have melanocytes present in the nail matrix and the nail bed. The numbers have not been studied; however, if they are scarcely found, they are not very melanin productive under normal conditions. If they are stimulated by Ultra Violet light in the A spectrum (PUVA), the melanocytes in the nail bed perform well and the patient's nail bed pigments readily (Fig. 8, Chapter 19). Thus, melanocytic lesions may accur in the matrix and in nail bed.

The melanocyte is found among the basal cells of the epithelium. Their number and behavior never interfere with the differentiation process of the keratinocytic population they cohabitate with, and only pigmentary characteristics are produced. Their cytologic and biologic characteristics are being studied; it is not presently known whether the melanocytes from the nail matrix and nail bed are different from that in glaborous skin.

Clinical lesions are formed: 1) By the increased activity in melanin production of the melanocyte, as seen in hormonal disturbances (Chapter 19); or 2) by the aggregation or proliferation of melanocytes which remain very restricted in the matrix and result in a continuous melanin deposit in the nail plate, clinically appearing as a longitudinal band, normally seen in the more pigmented races and less frequently in orientals. The number of studied cases of normal pigmented bands are so few, that doubt exists regarding the nature of the melanocytes seen in the basilar portion of the epithelium. There is question concerning whether it is it a junction nevus or melanocytic hyperplasia. As long as the clinical appearance of the final keratinocytic (stratum corneum) or onychocytic layer (nail plate) is intact (normal), it may be said that the lesion can be totally cured. All that it needs is a clinician which can recognize the lesion.

As the melanocyte's behavior proceeds in an abnormal pattern, it increases in numbers. Also, atypically, the point in time will be reached when abnormal melanocytes will interfere with the normal keratinization or differentiation process of the host keratinocytic layer and result in a dyskeratosis, manifested clinically as a scale. In the nail bed, this can be difficult to discern, but when it involves the matrix area it results in a defective nail plate which is easier to see. Thus, abnormalities in the thickness of the nail plate are an anonymous sign compared to only pigmentary changes.

Clinically, the following classification of melanocytic lesion can be seen:

1) Diffuse pigmentation of the nail unit (hormonal or drugs).
2) Discrete pigmented lesion of the nail matrix-nail plate, associated with similar lesions on the oral mucosa (Laugier-Hunziker).
3) Discrete pigmented longitudinal bands of the nail plate only (normal in darker races rarer in lighter ones).
4) Discrete macular lesions of the nail be (Junction Nevus?)
5) Discrete pigmented longitudinal bands appearing in caucasions in the 45-60 age group.

6) Acral Lentiginuous Melanoma.
7) Superficial Spreading Malignant Melanoma.
8) Nodular Melanoma.

The lesions of category 1, 2, and 3, are refered to in Chapter 19, "Pigmentation." Category 4, Macular pigmentation of nail bed, was described by Higachi, who believed these melanicyte nests to represent a junction nevus. It is still unknown whether these lesions progress in surface areas or if the condition is unique to orientals.

NOTES

1. Mikhail, G.R.: Bowen's disease and squamous cell carcinoma of the nail bed. *Arch. Derm. 110*: 267–270, 1974.

1a. Lupulescu, A., Pinkus, H., Birmingham, D.J., Usndek, H.E. and Posch, J.L.: Lentigo maligna of the fingertip. *Arch. Derm. 107*: 717–722, 1973.

2. Hoffman, S. Basal cell carcinoma of the nail bed *Arch. Derm. 108*: 828, 1973.

3. Shapiro, L. and Baraf, C.S.: Subungual epidermal carcinoma and keratoacanthoma. *Cancer 25*: 141–152, 1970.

4. Albom, M.J.: Squamous cell carcinoma of the finger and nail bed. *J. Derm. Surg. 1*: 2, 43–48. 1975.

5. Lamp, J.C., Graham, J.H., Urbach, F. and Burgoon, C.F.: Keratoacanthoma of the subungual region. *J. Bone and Joint Surgery 46A*: 1721–1731, 1964.

6. Macaulay, W.L.: Subungual Keratoacanthoma. *Arch. Derm. 112*: 1004–1005, 1976.

7. Hicks, M.C., Kalmon, E.J. Jr., and Glasser, S.M.: Metastatic malignancy to Phalanges, *Southern Med. Journ. 57*: 84–88, 1964.

8. Camiel, M.R., Aron, B.S., Alexander, L.L., Benninghoff, D.L. and Minkowitz, S.: Metastasis to palm, sole, nail bed, nose, face and scalp from unsuspected carcinoma of the lung. *Cancer 23*: 214–220, 1969.

9. Panebianco, A.C., Kaupp, H.A.: Bilateral thumb metastasis from breast carcinoma. *Arch Surg. 96*: 216–218, 1968.

10. Gottlieb, J.A. and Schermer, D.R.: Cutaneous metastasis from carcinoma of the colon. Letters to Editor. *JAMA 213*: 2083, 1970.

11. Clark, W.H., Bernardino, E.A., Reed, R.J., Kopf, A.W., "Acral Lentiginous Melanomas Including Melanomas of Mucous Membranes" chapter in *Human Melanoma: The Benign and Malignant Lesions and their Precursors,* W.H. Clark, M.J. Mastrangelo, L.I. Goldman. New York: Grune and Stratton, Inc., 1978.

12. Booher, R.H. and Pack, G.T. Malignant melanoma of the feet and hands. *Surgery 42*: 1085, 1957.

13. Decker, A.M. and Chaness, J.T., Melanocarcinoma of the Plantar surface of the foot. *Surgery*: 29, 731, 1951.

14. Nordlung, J.T., Clinical appearance of cutaneous melanomas. *Yale J. Biol. Med. 48*: 403, 1975.

15. Elwood, J.M. and Lee, J.A.H. Recent data on the epidemiology of malignant melanoma. *Semin. Oncol. 2*: 149, 1975.

16. Pack, G.T. and Davis, J. The relation of race and complexion to the incidence of moles and melanomas. *Ann. NY Acad. Sci. 100*: 719, 1963.

17. Arrington, J.H., Reed, R.J., Ichinose, H., Kremetz, E.T., Acral lentiginous melanoma—a distinctive variant of human cutaneous malignant melanoma. *Am. J. Surg. Path. 1*: 2131, 1977.

Index